Teleophthalmology in Preventive Medicine

Teleophthalmology in Preventive Medicine

Georg Michelson

Editor

Teleophthalmology in Preventive Medicine

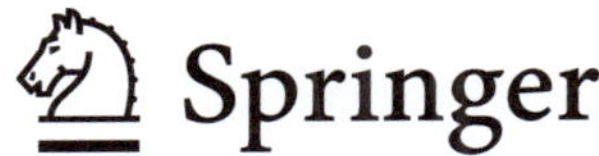

Editor
Georg Michelson
Department of Ophthalmology
University Erlangen-Nürnberg
Erlangen, Germany

ISBN 978-3-662-52310-0   ISBN 978-3-662-44975-2   (eBook)
DOI 10.1007/978-3-662-44975-2
Springer Berlin Heidelberg New York Dordrecht London

Preface

One important aim of future medicine should be to detect diseases at a stage when there are only minor or no manifestations of its symptoms. In such cases, an early therapy can avoid severe consequences of the disease and extend the lifetime without deficits in function. This type of medicine is called preventive medicine.

In olden times, the eye was considered a gateway to medical wisdom.

The evaluation of the retina and optic nerve head might be an important cornerstone in preventive medicine. The vasculature, the neurons and axons of the retina, and the optic nerve show early symptoms of some systemic diseases like arterial hypertension and diabetes and neurodegenerative diseases like Alzheimer's. Retinal cells, neurons, and vessels serve as well-evidenced surrogate parameters for early detection of diseases, predicting the risk of fatal events and monitoring the effect of therapy.

As the retina is very well accessible by novel optical methods, morphological and functional changes become visible in early stages of systemic diseases.

Tele-ophthalmology involves imaging of the retina and the optic nerve of patients from remote locations combined with a telemedical assessment of these images by expert ophthalmologists using computer-aided image analysis systems. The benefit of tele-ophthalmology is that it involves transport of only data and images and does not require the transport of subjects.

Thus, tele-ophthalmology might become an important tool for providers of preventive medicine to detect early signs of systemic diseases related to metabolism, vessels, and neuronal tissues. Early knowledge of changes in the retina helps to evaluate the risk of severe diseases and to adopt a suitable therapy.

In addition, tele-ophthalmology can be used to screen people for vision-threatening diseases like AMD, glaucoma, and trachoma. Early therapy in AMD, diabetic retinopathy, and glaucoma reduces the risk of visual impairment.

To be most effective, tele-ophthalmology should use latest technologies in imaging and information processing.

The overall aim of this book is to describe (1) clinical applications of tele-ophthalmology and (2) novel methods used in tele-ophthalmology by experts in the field.

The book *Tele-Ophthalmology in Preventive Medicine* targets medical care providers interested in tele-ophthalmology.

The book gives an overview of medical applications, methods, and novel technologies in tele-ophthalmology especially in the area of preventive medicine. It also gives future prospects for methods of detecting early signs of neurodegenerative diseases in the retina and describes innovative projects of interdisciplinary cooperation in preventive medicine. In addition, a major part of the book is devoted to novel imaging methods and latest information technologies like mobile communication and Web 2.0 applications in tele-ophthalmology.

Erlangen, Germany   Georg Michelson, MD

Contents

Contributors

Michael David Abràmoff, MD, PhD Retina Service, Department of Ophthalmology and Visual Sciences, Department of Electrical and Computer Engineering, Department of Biomedical Engineering, Iowa City Veterans Medical Center, University of Iowa, Iowa City, IA, USA

Werner Adler, PhD Department of of Medical Informatics, Biometry and Epidemiology, Friedrich-Alexander University Erlangen-Nuremberg, Erlangen, Germany

Rüdiger Bock Pattern Recognition Lab, Department of Computer Science, Friedrich-Alexander-Universität Erlangen Nürnberg, Erlangen, Bavaria, Germany

Erlangen Graduate School in Advanced Optical Technologies (SAOT), Erlangen, Germany

Bernhard Höher, Dipl.-Ing Institute of Microwaves and Photonics, University of Erlangen Nuremberg, Erlangen, Germany

Lehrstuhl für Hochfrequenztechnik, Erlangen, Germany

Folkert K. Horn, PhD Department of Ophthalmology, University Medical Center Erlangen, Erlangen, Germany

Department of Ophthalmology, University Eye Hospital, Friedrich-Alexander University Erlangen-Nürnberg, Erlangen, Germany

Universitäts-Augenklinik, Erlangen, Germany

Joachim Hornegger, PhD-Ing. Pattern Recognition Lab, Department of Computer Science, Friedrich-Alexander-Universität Erlangen Nürnberg, Erlangen, Bavaria, Germany

Erlangen Graduate School in Advanced Optical Technologies (SAOT), Erlangen, Germany

David Huang, MD, PhD Casey Eye Institute, Oregon Health & Science University, Portland, OR, USA

Yali Jia, PhD Casey Eye Institute, Oregon Health & Science University, Portland, OR, USA

Simon Kaja, PhD Department of Ophthalmology, Vision Research Center, University of Missouri-Kansas City School of Medicine, Kansas City, MO, USA

K&P Scientific LLC, Kansas City, MO, USA

Yogesan Kanagasingam, PhD The Australian e-Health Research Centre, CCI, CSIRO, Floreat, Australia

Thomas Kohler, MSc Pattern Recognition Lab, Department of Computer Science, Friedrich-Alexander-Universität Erlangen Nürnberg, Erlangen, Bavaria, Germany

Erlangen Graduate School in Advanced Optical Technologies (SAOT), Erlangen, Germany

Georg Michelson, MD Department of Ophthalmology, Interdisciplinary Center of Ophthalmic Preventive Medicine and Imaging, Friedrich-Alexander University Erlangen-Nürnberg, Erlangen, Germany

Verlag ONJOPH.COM, Erlangen, Germany

Erlangen Graduate School in Advanced Optical Technologies (SAOT), Erlangen, Germany

Moritz Michelson Verlag ONJOPH.COM, Erlangen, Germany

Yuliya Naumchuk, BS Department of Ophthalmology, Vision Research Center, University of Missouri-Kansas City School of Medicine, Kansas City, MO, USA

Meindert Niemeijer, PhD IDx, LLC, Iowa City, IA, USA

Department of Ophthalmology and Visual SciencesThe University of Iowa Hospitals and Clinics, Iowa City, IA, USA

Michel Paques, MD, PhDmichel.paques@gmail.com Clinical Investigation Center 503, Quinze-Vingts Hospital, University Pierre et Marie Curie-Paris6, Paris, France

Bernhard Schmauss, PhD.-Ing Institute of Microwaves and Photonics, University of Erlangen Nuremberg, Erlangen, Germany

Vinay A. Shah, MD Dean McGee Eye Institute, University of Oklahoma, Oklahoma City, OK, USA

Peter Voigtmann, Dipl.-Kfm Voigtmann GmbH, Nürnberg, Germany

Johannes Wolz Department of Ophthalmology, University Hospital of the Friedrich-Alexander-University Erlangen-Nürnberg, Erlangen, Germany

Di Xiao, PhD The Australian e-Health Research Centre, CCI, CSIRO, Floreat, Australia

Prevalence of Retinal Microangiopathic Abnormalities and Optic Nerve Atrophy in Normotensive, Nondiabetic, "Healthy" Subjects Gained by a Retina Check of the Tele-ophthalmic Consultation Service Talkingeyes®

Georg Michelson and Johannes Wolz

Contents

G. Michelson, MD (✉)
Department of Ophthalmology, Interdisciplinary
Center of Ophthalmic Preventive Medicine
and Imaging, Friedrich-Alexander University
Erlangen-Nürnberg, Schwabachanlage 6,
Erlangen D-91054, Germany
e-mail: Georg.michelson@uk-erlangen.de

J. Wolz
Department of Ophthalmology, University Hospital
of the Friedrich-Alexander-University
Erlangen-Nürnberg, Erlangen, Germany

1.1   Background

The unique structure-function correlations make the anterior visual pathway with retina and optic nerve an ideal model for investigating diseases that target microangiopathies, axonal and neuronal degeneration.

Abnormalities of the optic nerve and the retinal microvascular bed, such as optic nerve atrophy, focal and generalized arteriolar narrowing and arteriovenous nicking, have been found as typical abnormalities of the ocular fundus in patients with systemic hypertension, diabetes or stroke [1, 2]. It is well known that retinal microvascular abnormalities are strongly related to past and current hypertension or diabetes mellitus.

Axonal and neuronal degeneration of the retina and optic nerve head is often observed in patients with systemic diseases or cerebral neurodegeneration. Retinal nerve fibre layer (RNFL) thickness is statistically reduced in patients with mild cognitive impairment, mild Alzheimer disease compared to controls. The retinal nerve fibre layer (RNFL) thickness followed by optic nerve atrophy is involved early during the course of amnestic mild cognitive impairment.

"Simple" optic nerve atrophy, arteriolar narrowing and arteriovenous nicking were also found

G. Michelson (ed.), *Teleophthalmology in Preventive Medicine*,
DOI 10.1007/978-3-662-44975-2_1, © Springer-Verlag Berlin Heidelberg 2015

in normotensive and nondiabetic populations. The origin of these changes in normotensive or nondiabetic subjects is not fully understood, but is favoured by several factors, including elevated blood lipids, smoking and lack of exercise. Previous studies have shown that arteriolar narrowing and arteriovenous nicking are related to increasing age. This was documented in mixed populations containing hypertensive and/or diabetic subjects.

In our study we investigated the prevalence of focal arteriolar narrowing, focal and generalized arteriolar narrowing, arteriovenous nicking and optic nerve atrophy in a group of nondiabetic, normotensive subjects without any systemic or ocular disease. The Tele-ophthalmic Consultation Service Talkingeyes® performed the photography of the posterior pole and the documentation of reported relevant information of existing ophthalmic, internal or neurological diseases. The tele-ophthalmic evaluation of retina and optic nerve head morphology was performed by an experienced eye doctor. The service was performed in institutions without ophthalmic expertise (Table 1.1).

1.2 Purpose

To examine the prevalence of "simple" optic nerve atrophy, retinal microvascular narrowing and arteriovenous nicking in a normotensive, nondiabetic, "healthy" population gained by the Tele-Ophthalmic Consultation Service Talkingeyes®.

1.3 Methods

1.3.1 Study Population

This report is based on examinations of over 9,400 men and women gained by the Tele-Ophthalmic Consultation Service Talkingeyes® [3–7] within the years 2007–2012. All participants underwent a profound interview documenting information of general medical, ocular medical and family history. By this interview age, gender, presence of arterial hypertension,

diabetes mellitus or any other systemic disease (such as kidney damages, cardiac infarction, coronary artery bypass) and incident stroke were reported.

For the analysis we selected $N=1,662$ "healthy" individuals aged 41–90 years without arterial hypertension, diabetes mellitus or any other systemic or ocular disease or stroke or heart infarction in medical history. Patients with nicotine abuse, with one eye missing or with retinal images that were not evaluable due to the poor image quality were excluded. $N=785$ participants were male (47 %), while $N=877$ were female (53 %). The age ranged from 41 to 89 years.

Systemic hypertension was defined as reported systolic blood pressure higher than 140 mmHg or a diastolic blood pressure higher than 90 mmHg and/or taking antihypertensive medication. Blood pressure values were documented as reported values. Diabetes was defined as reported HbA1c value higher than 6 % and/or taking antidiabetic medication.

1.3.2 Procedures

The telemedical evaluation by the Tele-Ophthalmic Consultation Service Talkingeyes® was validated by comparing the diagnoses gained by the telemedical approach versus a regular ophthalmological examination with dilated pupils [8, 9].

The Tele-Ophthalmic Consultation Service Talkingeyes® served as virtual telemedical consultant in institutions without ophthalmic expertise documenting general and ocular medical history, visual function and retina and optic nerve head morphology. The used software (MedStage, Siemens, Talkingeyes and more) is browser-independent running at PC, tablets and smartphones. All imaging techniques can be used.

In this study digital retinal images of both eyes were taken with a 45° non-mydriatic colour fundus camera (KOWA NM-45, non-mydriatic-alpha) centred on the papilla of the optic nerve (Fig. 1.1). Pupils were not dilated. After completing the medical interview (Tables 1.2, 1.3, 1.4 and 1.5), selected clinical images of the

Table 1.1 The age dependency of retinal microvascular abnormalities in a nondiabetic, normotensive, "healthy" population

Age (years)	Focal arteriolar narrowing		Generalized art. narrowing		Arteriovenous nicking		Optic nerve atrophy	
	n/N	Prevalence %	n/N	Prevalence %	n/N	Prevalence %	n/N	Prevalence %
41–50	55/509	10.8	18/509	3.5	10/509	2.0	4/509	0.8
51–60	104/577	18.0	26/577	4.5	20/577	3.5	13/577	2.3
61–70	123/383	32.1	34/383	8.9	25/383	6.5	13/383	3.4
71–80	59/160	36.9	14/160	8.8	13/160	8.1	16/160	10.0
81–90	12/33	36.4	5/33	15.2	3/33	9.1	5/33	15.2
		$P=0.037*$		$P=0.071$		$P=0.017*$		$P=0.017*$
		$R^2=0.963$		$R^2=0.929$		$R^2=0.983$		$R^2=0.983$
All ages	**353/1,662**	**21.2**	**97/1,662**	**5.8**	**71/1,662**	**4.3**	**51/1,662**	**3.1**

Reprinted with permission from Talkingeyes&more GmbH
* <0.05

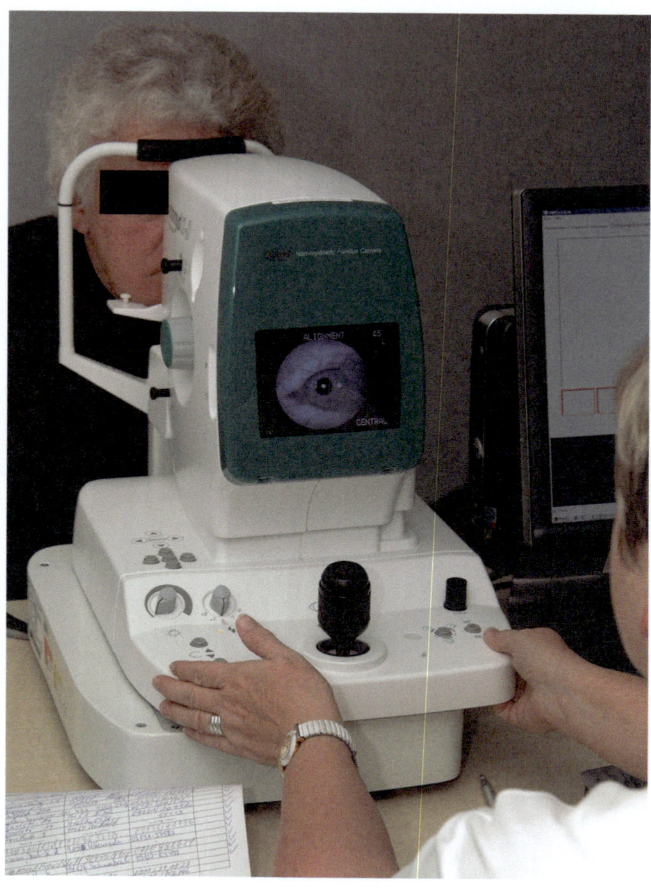

Fig. 1.1 Image acquisition by a non-mydriatic fundus camera (Reprinted with permission from Talkingeyes&more GmbH)

Table 1.2 MedStage: date entry of a new patient

Enter new participant data

PERSON			CONTACT		
Salutation	Mr. ▾		Language for communication	english ▾	
Last Name	Test		Phone (daytime)		
First Name	Test		Phone (evening)		
Date of birth (DD/MM/YYYY)	22.11.2000		Email		
Year of birth			Login	test.test	
Street	street		Password	4Y2rm2zAgw	
Postcode	99999		Email when result is ready?	no ▾	
City	city		Result delivery	Internet download ▾	
Country	country				

Reprinted with permission from Talkingeyes&more GmbH

Table 1.3 MedStage: general medical history part I

Registration	**Medical History 1/3**

SLOTS

Next appointments — Test Test ▼

Tasklist — Standard ▼

1. Age and Gender

Date of birth (DD/MM/YYYY)   22/11/2000

Gender   male ▼

2. Coronary Heart Diseases (CHD)

Cardiac infarction   no ▼   in year: [ ]

Balloon angioplasty   no ▼   in year: [ ]

Bypass surgery   no ▼   in year: [ ]

3. Stroke

Did patient suffer a stroke?   no ▼   in year: [ ]

4. Carotid Surgery

Did patient have a carotid surgery?   no ▼   in year: [ ]

5. Stress-related problems

in the chest   no ▼

Constrictive chest pain and shortness of breath during physical exertion or angina pectoris

in the legs   no ▼

Atherosclerosis in the legs, peripheral arterial disease (PAD)

6. Blood Pressure

What is the patient's blood pressure?   [ ] / [ ] mmHg

7. Hypertension

Does patient suffer from raised blood pressure?   no ▼   since: [ ]

If yes, start of treatment for hypertension   [ ]

Medication to lower blood pressure   [ ]

8. Blood Sugar (Glucose)

Does patient suffer from raised blood sugar?   no ▼   since: [ ]

If yes, start of treatment for diabetes   [ ]

What is the patient's HbA1c level?   [ ] %

Complications of diabetes   --- ▼   since: [ ]

Diabetic retinopathy   --- ▼   since: [ ]

Polyneuropathy   --- ▼   since: [ ]

Kidney diseases   --- ▼   since: [ ]

Reprinted with permission from Talkingeyes&more GmbH

anterior, the posterior segment or other modalities were uploaded in the electronic patient chart (Table 1.6) followed by a telemedical evaluation by an experienced eye doctor. Tables 1.2, 1.3, 1.4 and 1.5 depict the data entry formulas and Table 1.6 the formula to upload images. All images were stored on a server using the web-based software MedStage. The medical evaluation of the colour fundus images and other images was done through telemedical analysis (Fig. 1.2). Figure 1.2 showed the standardized procedure of the medical evaluation. Each fundus image was evaluated by an experienced ophthalmologist using a standardized protocol with defined criteria, namely, focal arteriolar narrowing, focal and generalized arteriolar narrowing, arteriovenous nicking and optic nerve atrophy. The evaluation of the images was facilitated by the options to zoom the images and to examine them in different aspects (colour image, red-free image and green channel image). "Simple" optic nerve atrophy was defined as a partly or

Table 1.4 MedStage: general medical history part II

Registration	Medical History 1/3	**Medical History 2/3**

Next appointments Test Test ▾

Tasklist Standard ▾

9. Cholesterol and Triglycerides

Raised cholesterol no ▾ since ☐

Raised level of blood fat no ▾ since ☐

If yes, start of treatment (cholesterol, triglycerides) ☐

Medication to lower cholesterol/triglycerides level ☐

Total cholesterol level ☐ mg/dl

LDL cholesterol level ☐ mg/dl

HDL cholesterol level ☐ mg/dl

Triglyceride level ☐ mg/dl

10. Smoking

Is patient smoker? no ▾

If yes, how much? ☐ cig./day since: ☐

11. Height, Weight and Waist Circumference

Height 200 cm **Weight** 100 kg

Waist circumference 100 cm

12. Physical Activity / Sports

How often does patient exercise? ☐ times per week

13. Eyeglasses

Does patient wear eyeglasses/lenses? no ▾

Refraction right (OD) ☐ dpt left (OS) ☐ dpt

14. Known Eye Diseases

Raised intraocular pressure no ▾

Macula degeneration no ▾

Other ☐

15. Family History

Diseases with relatives

Cardiac infarction or stroke
Raised intraocular pressure (glaucoma)
Senile dementia

☐ grandparents

☐ parents

☐ siblings

☐ children

Reprinted with permission from Talkingeyes&more GmbH

completely atrophic optic nerve head with a pale rim, but no cupping.

The tele-ophthalmological evaluation was performed within three working days, in case of emergency within 2 h. The medical report was available by html- or pdf-format by the medical doctor or by the patient using ID and a password. Figure 1.3 depicts the scheme of the complete procedure.

Table 1.5 MedStage: ocular medical history and visual acuity, IOP

Medical history of the eyes

Good vision as child	yes
First glasses in age	---
Strabism	no in year:
Comment on "Strabism"	
Eye surgery	no in year:
Comment on "Eye surgery"	
Laser	no in year:
Comment on "Laser"	
Eye trauma	no in year:
Comment on "Eye trauma"	
Glaucoma	no in year:
Comment on "Glaucoma"	
Retinal detachment	no in year:
Comment on "Retinal detachment"	
Inflammation (Uveitis)	no in year:
Comment on "Inflammation (Uveitis)"	
Deterioration of vision	no in year:
Comment on "Deterioration of vision"	
Eye drops	--- since:
Comment on "Eye drops"	

Visual acuity

	right (OD)	left (OS)
Correction	unknown	
Visual acuity	unknown	unknown
Contrast sensitivity	unknown	unknown
Stereo vision / Disparity in arc sec	---	
Disparity method	unknown	

Autorefraction

	right (OD)	left (OS)
spherical	unknown	unknown
cylindrical	unknown	unknown
axis	unknown	unknown

Refraction of glasses

	right (OD)	left (OS)
spherical	unknown	unknown
cylindrical	unknown	unknown
axis	unknown	unknown

Difference Autorefraction and Glasses

	right (OD)	left (OS)

Intraoccular pressure

	right (OD)	left (OS)
Method	unknown	unknown
IOP value in mmHg	unknown	unknown

Other examinations

Pupillary distance (PD) in mm	unknown

Reprinted with permission from Talkingeyes&more GmbH

Table 1.6 MedStage: upload of images examination number: FAU-2014-01-10-01-TT

Examination Number: FAU-2014-01-10-01-TT

Important notice: *You can upload only images of type PNG (24 bit color images with lossless compression) or JPEG (24 bit color images with lossy compression)!*

Images RIGHT Eye (OD)	Images LEFT Eye (OS)
Fundus images - Right eye (OD)	**Fundus images - Left eye (OS)**
1st fundus image — Not yet uploaded — Upload image …	1st fundus image — Not yet uploaded — Upload image …
2nd fundus image — Not yet uploaded — Upload image …	2nd fundus image — Not yet uploaded — Upload image …
3rd fundus image — Upload image … — Not yet uploaded	3rd fundus image — Upload image … — Not yet uploaded
Images anterior segment - Right eye (OD) — Upload image …	**Images anterior segment - Left eye (OS)** — Upload image …
Other eye images (OCT, Angiogram, …) - Right Eye (OD) — Upload image … — Upload image … — Upload image … — Upload image … — Upload image …	**Other eye images (OCT, Angiogram, …) - Left eye (OS)** — Upload image … — Upload image … — Upload image … — Upload image … — Upload image …

Finalize and release images for assessment - after this step, no more images can be added.

Back - further images may be added later.

Reprinted with permission from Talkingeyes&more GmbH

1.3.3 Statistical Analysis

Statistical analysis was performed with SPSS Vol. 20.0 and 21.0. We divided the study group into decades of age (41–50 years, 51–60 years, 61–70 years, 71–80 years, 81–90 years). The prevalence of optic nerve atrophy, focal arteriolar narrowing, focal and generalized arteriolar narrowing, arteriovenous nicking, retinal microinfarcts and retinal haemorrhages was calculated

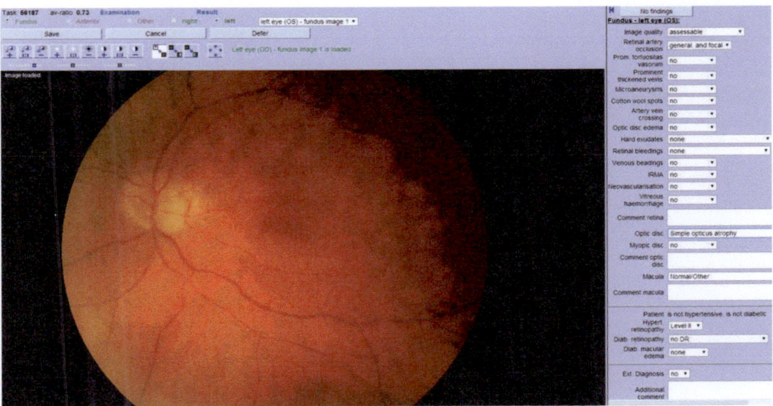

Fig. 1.2 Standardized medical evaluation of a fundus image (Reprinted with permission from Talkingeyes&more GmbH)

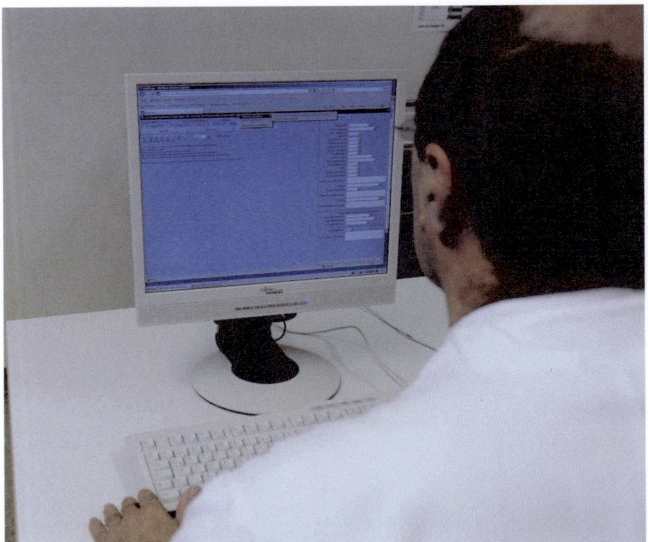

Fig. 1.3 Scheme of complete telemedical procedure (data and image acquisition, tele-ophthalmological evaluation, report generation) (Reprinted with permission from Talkingeyes&more GmbH)

for each decade. A square regression model was used to find a correlation between the prevalence of retinal microvascular abnormalities and age. For the analysis only the evaluation of the image of the right eye was used.

1.4   Results

In the examined group we found no retinal micro-infarcts or retinal haemorrhages. The prevalence of focal narrowing, generalized narrowing, arteriovenous nicking and optic nerve atrophy in healthy subjects is strongly age related. Figure 1.4

shows the age dependencies. The correlation coefficients were for optic nerve atrophy $R2=0.983$ ($p=0.017$), generalized arteriolar narrowing $R2=0.92$ ($p=0.07$), focal arteriolar narrowing $R2=0.963$ ($p=0.037$) and arteriovenous nicking $R2=0.983$ ($p=0.017$). The prevalence of optic nerve atrophy rose from 0.8 % in the 4th decade to 15.2 % in the 8th decade (factor 19), the prevalence of generalized arteriolar narrowing from 3.5 % in the 4th decade to 15.2 % in the 8th decade (factor 4.3), the prevalence of focal arteriolar narrowing from 10 % in the 4th decade to 36 % in the 8th decade (factor 3.6) and the prevalence of arteriovenous nicking from 2 % in

Fig. 1.4 The prevalence of "simple" optic nerve atrophy and retinal microvascular abnormalities in healthy subjects by decades

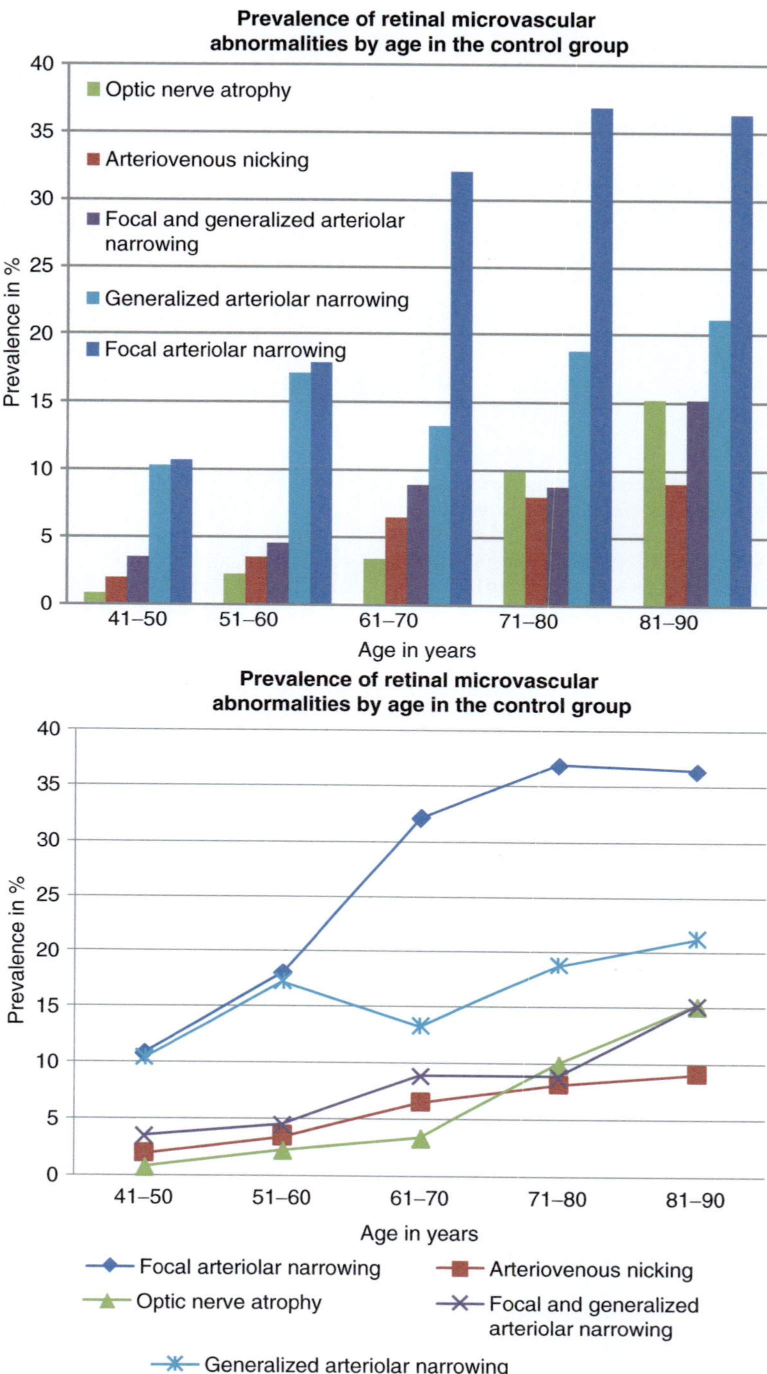

the 4th decade to 9 % in the 8th decade(factor 4.5). Table 1.1 shows detailed information about the prevalence of focal arteriolar narrowing, focal and generalized narrowing, arteriovenous nicking and optic nerve atrophy by decades. The age dependency of optic nerve atrophy, arteriovenous nicking and focal arteriolar narrowing was significant at $p < 0.05$.

1.5 Discussion

The technique used by the Tele-Ophthalmic Consultation Service Talkingeyes® to diagnose telemedically optic nerve atrophy or abnormalities of retinal vessels was validated by a comparative observational study including $N=47$ hypertensive and/or diabetic subjects. In this study the fundus was judged ophthalmoscopically and subsequently by the telemedical approach. The reliability of the two diagnostic methods was then calculated. The largest concordance of the two diagnosis methods was achieved, in descending order, for stage of hypertensive retinopathy, retinal bleeding, stage of diabetic retinopathy and the optic nerve head findings. It was concluded that the tele-ophthalmic approach achieved good results as compared to the ophthalmoscopic judgement in relation to retinopathy assessment criteria [10, 11].

1.5.1 Optic Nerve Atrophy

In the presented study we found a prevalence of optic nerve atrophy in 0.8 % of normotensive, nondiabetic, "healthy" subjects aged 41–50 years and a prevalence up to 15.2 % in subjects aged 81–90 years.

In the literature there is no data about the prevalence of optic nerve atrophy in healthy subjects. Only prevalences of microangiopathic lesions and glaucomatous optic nerve atrophy in healthy subjects were reported [8, 9, 12, 13]. In a former study of our group [8], we examined telemedically in 19.294 Caucasians the retina and the optic nerve head in respect to microangiopathic changes and glaucomatous optic nerve atrophy using the above-described technique. Glaucomatous optic nerve atrophy was diagnosed when specific glaucomatous morphological alterations of the optic nerve head were present. In this study the reported prevalence of glaucomatous optic nerve atrophy in the different age groups was 0.07 % (45–49 years), 0.40 % (50–54 years), 0.45 % (55–59 years) and 0.82 % (60–64 years) [9]. Comparing the found prevalence of "simple" optic nerve atrophy with the reported prevalence of glaucomatous optic nerve atrophy, the prevalence of "simple" optic nerve atrophy is lower by factor 10.

1.5.2 Retinal Microangiopathic Abnormalities

In the Beaver Dam Eye Study, the Atherosclerosis Risk in Communities Study and the Cardiovascular Health Study, prevalences of microangiopathic changes in healthy subjects were reported.

We found in healthy normals a prevalence of 4.3 % of arteriovenous nicking. In the Beaver Dam Eye Study, nondiabetic subjects including hypertensive individuals with a mean age of 62 years were examined. In this study Klein et al. investigated a cohort of 4,311 nondiabetic individuals aged 43–84 years [14, 15]. Retinal images were taken with a 30° stereoscopic colour fundus camera centred on the optic disc and the macula and additionally with a non-stereoscopic colour fundus camera focusing temporal to but including the fovea of each eye [16]. They found in normotensive subjects focal narrowing in 11 % and arteriovenous nicking in 2 %.

In the Atherosclerosis Risk in Communities Study, 8,772 nondiabetic subjects including hypertensive individuals aged from 51 to 72 years with a mean age of 59.5 years were examined. Pictures of 8.772 individuals [17] which included hypertensive subjects were assessed in their analysis. For retinal imaging a 45° fundus camera was used and centred between the optic disc and macula of one randomly selected eye [18–20]. They found in normotensive subjects focal narrowing in 4.5 % and arteriovenous nicking in 4.6 %.

In the Cardiovascular Health Study, 2,050 nondiabetic subjects including hypertensive individuals with a mean age of 78.5 years were examined. In this study, a cohort of 2,050 nondiabetic subjects aged 69–97 years was examined, including hypertensive individuals and a small group of stroke patients [21]. Retinal photographs were taken with a 45° fundus camera from one randomly selected eye and centred between the optic disc and macula. They found in normotensive subjects focal narrowing in 6.1 % and arteriovenous nicking in 5.9 %.

We found similar results. In our study the prevalence of arteriovenous nicking was 4.3 %, compared to 2 % in the Beaver Dam Eye Study, 4.6 % in the Atherosclerosis Risk in Communities Study and 5.9 % in the Cardiovascular Health Study. In focal narrowing our data differ from published data from other groups. We found a prevalence of focal arteriolar narrowing in 21 % of nondiabetic, normotensive, "healthy" subjects. The higher prevalence of focal arteriolar narrowing found in our study compared with the results of previous studies may be due to a higher average age in our study group and a different grading of the retinal images. The differences might be caused by higher mean ages.

Conclusion

The tele-ophthalmic technique Talkingeyes® allowed the telemedical evaluation of the anterior part of the visual pathway using data of the medical history, visual function and images of the retina and optic nerve head morphology. We found that the prevalence of microvascular alterations and optic nerve atrophy in healthy subjects was strongly age related. The prevalences of retinal microangiopathic changes in the retina and optic nerve head in different decades of age ranged for focal narrowing from 10 to 36 %, for generalized narrowing from 3 to 15 %, for arteriovenous nicking from 2 to 9 % and for "simple" optic nerve atrophy from 0.8 to 15 %. Thus, a telemedical evaluation of patient in respect to optic nerve pathology or microangiopathic changes should refer to age-related prevalences of healthy controls.

References

1. Wong TY, Mitchell P. Hypertensive retinopathy. N Engl J Med. 2004;351:2311.
2. De Silva DA, Manzano JJF, Liu EY, et al. Retinal microvascular changes and subsequent vascular events after ischemic stroke. Neurol. 2011;77(9):896–903
3. Michelson G, Groh M, Groh MJ, Baleanu D, Harazny J, Horstmann R, Kolominsky-Rabas P. Telemedical-supported screening of retinal vessels ("talking eyes"). Klin Monbl Augenheilkd. 2005;222(4):319–25. German.
4. Michelson G. TalkingEyes-and-more. Biomed Tech (Berl). 2005;50(7–8):218–26. German.
5. Händel A, Jünemann AG, Prokosch HU, Beyer A, Ganslandt T, Grolik R, Klein A, Mrosek A, Michelson G, Kruse FE. Web-based electronic patient record as an instrument for quality assurance within an integrated care concept. Klin Monbl Augenheilkd. 2009;226(3):161–7.
6. Schargus M, Michelson G, Grehn F. Electronic patient records and teleophthalmology: part 1: introduction to the various systems and standards. Ophthalmologe. 2011;108(5):473–84. doi:10.1007/s00347-010-2314-5. German.
7. Schargus M, Michelson G, Grehn F. Electronic patient records and teleophthalmology. Part 2: concrete projects in ophthalmology. Ophthalmologe. 2011;108(7):687–95. doi:10.1007/s00347-011-2353-6; quiz 696. German.
8. Adler W, Wärntges S, Lausen B, Michelson G. Prevalence of glaucomatous optic nerve atrophy among a working population in Germany diagnosed by a telemedical approach. Klin Monbl Augenheilkd. 2010;227(11):905–11.
9. Bock R, Meier J, Nyúl LG, Hornegger J, Michelson G. Glaucoma risk index: automated glaucoma detection from color fundus images. Med Image Anal. 2010;14(3):471–81.
10. Michelson G, Engelhorn T, Dörfler A. Retinal microangiopathy in arterial hypertension as an early marker of a cerebral macroangiopathy. Dtsch Med Wochenschr. 2011;136(46):2355–8. doi:10.1055/s-0031-1292050. Epub 2011 Nov 8. German.
11. Huchzermeyer C, Schaller B, Schmid K, Schmieder RE, Michelson G. Comparison of early retinal microvascular changes and microalbuminuria as indicators for increased cardiovascular risk. Klin Monbl Augenheilkd. 2011;228(11):1003–8.
12. Chrástek R, Wolf M, Donath K, Niemann H, Paulus D, Hothorn T, Lausen B, Lämmer R, Mardin CY, Michelson G. Automated segmentation of the optic nerve head for diagnosis of glaucoma. Med Image Anal. 2005;9(4):297–314.
13. Michelson G, Wärntges S, Hornegger J, Lausen B. The papilla as screening parameter for early diagnosis of glaucoma. Dtsch Arztebl Int. 2008;105(34–35):583–9.
14. Klein R. Retinopathy in a population based study. Trans Am Ophthalmol Soc. 1992;90:567.
15. Klein R, Klein BEK, Moss SE, Wang Q. Hypertension and retinopathy, arteriolar narrowing, arteriovenous nicking in a population. Arch Ophthalmol. 1994;112:92–8.

16. Klein R, Klein BEK, Tomany SC, Wong TY. The relation of retinal microvascular characteristics to age-related eye disease: the Beaver Dam eye study. Am J Ophthalmol. 2004;137:436.

17. Klein R, Sharrett AR, Klein BEK, et al. Are retinal arteriolar abnormalities related to atherosclerosis? The Atherosclerosis Risk in Communities Study. Arterioscler Thromb Vasc Biol. 2000;20:1644.

18. Hubbard LD, Brothers RJ, King WN, et al. Methods for evaluation of retinal microvascular abnormalities associated with hypertension/sclerosis in the Atherosclerosis Risk in Communities Study. Ophthalmology. 1999;106:2271.

19. Klein R, Sharrett AR, Klein BEK, et al. Are retinal arteriolar abnormalities related to atherosclerosis? The Atherosclerosis Risk in Communities Study. Arterioscler Thromb Vasc Biol. 2000;20:1645.

20. Wong TY, Klein R, Couper DJ, et al. Retinal microvascular abnormalities and incident stroke: the Atherosclerosis Risk in Communities Study. Lancet. 2001;358:1135.

21. Wong TY, Klein R, Sharrett AR, et al. The prevalence and risk factors of retinal microvascular abnormalities in older persons. The Cardiovascular Health Study. Am Acad Ophthalmol. 2003;110:659.

Screening of the Retina in Diabetes Patients by Morphological Means

Di Xiao and Yogesan Kanagasingam

Contents

D. Xiao, PhD • Y. Kanagasingam, PhD (✉)
The Australian e-Health Research Centre,
DPAS, CSIRO, 65 Brockway Rd,
Floreat, WA 6014, Australia
e-mail: xia020@csiro.au; kan063@csiro.au

2.1 Diabetic Retinopathy and Its Prevalence

Diabetic retinopathy (DR), one of the major and long-term microvascular complications of diabetes, is the most common cause of vision loss and blindness in the working-age adults in industrialized countries. DR has been independently associated with increased mortality [1], heart disease [2], and kidney disorders [3]. It is well established that the onset and progression of DR are significantly associated with three key risk factors: longer duration of diabetes, poor glycemic control and increased blood pressure. The World Health Organization (WHO) announced that 347 million people worldwide had diabetes in 2012 and in 2030, diabetes will be the 7th leading cause of death [4]. With the increased prevalence of Type 1, and especially Type 2 diabetes, it is anticipated that the impact of vision impairment and blindness associated with DR will invariably increase in the coming decades.

On the other hand, diabetic retinopathy is a treatable disease throughout its progression. Though it is irreversible, the blindness risk can be reduced by early DR recognition, routine referral, regular follow-up examination and prompt treatment. According to the WHO, evidence-based treatment can significantly reduce the risk for blindness, and clinical studies have also shown that appropriate treatment can reduce it by more than 90 % [5]. Especially for diabetic macular oedema (DME), early intervention can

G. Michelson (ed.), *Teleophthalmology in Preventive Medicine*,
DOI 10.1007/978-3-662-44975-2_2, © Springer-Verlag Berlin Heidelberg 2015

significantly reduce severe visual loss by 50 % at 5 years. According to the recommendation from the WHO, diabetes patients should take annual eye examination for promising early-stage diagnosis of DR.

For society, the cost of diabetes management is a big burden. It is estimated the number of diabetes patients will increase to 44.1 million. The diabetes-related health expenditure will achieve up to US$171 billion [6, 7]. Therefore, early-stage DR detection and treatment based on guideline-recommended care will not only benefit patients but also reduce the economic burdens on society.

Timely diagnosis and evidence-based treatment for diabetes patients are important for preventing vision loss. However, the current society faces the conflict of increasing number of diabetics and decreasing number of ophthalmologists. Traditional eye fundus examination using ophthalmoscope or biomicroscopy must be conducted in clinics by ophthalmologists or in an acute eye care service model, which is difficult to be extended for DR prevention. And how to approach remote or rural areas which lack ophthalmologists is another issue.

In the past decade, there is a general agreement that digital colour fundus photography has obvious advantages compared to traditional ophthalmoscopy in diabetic retinopathy diagnosis. Digital fundus images are easy for storage and transmission and, therefore, can facilitate remote DR diagnosis. And with the rapid development of telemedicine and telehealth, digital fundus imaging and image-based diagnosis can be easily combined with the telehealth service model for expanding the service area of ophthalmologists that traditional approaches cannot reach. Therefore, tele-ophthalmology could be a potential and cost-effective method for eye care and DR-related service.

This chapter will focus on colour fundus image-based DR detection and DR screening by morphological features from the images and introduce the current progress of DR screening programmes based on colour fundus image grading.

2.2 DR Pathological Features on Colour Fundus Images

Diabetic retinopathy usually causes damage to microvascular vessels in the retina and further causes bleeding and fluid leakage.

Microaneurysms (MAs) present in the retina due to high sugar levels in the blood and are swellings of capillaries caused by capillary occlusion and vessel wall weakening. On colour fundus images, MAs morphologically appear as small roughly circular red objects with consistent size. They have similar pixel intensity (colour) to the blood vessels. MAs are the earliest symptom of DR disease.

Haemorrhages (HMs) are caused from abnormal bleeding, meaning an ischaemic retina (loss of oxygen). On a colour fundus image, HMs' pixel intensity is similar as that of blood vessels. The haemorrhages in their morphological shapes can appear as dot-and-blot HMs or large HMs. Large retinal haemorrhages (as flame-shaped HMs) are usually caused by abnormally fragile retinal blood vessels and represent a symptom of advanced disease. If HMs appear at the macular region, they may interfere with vision. When a vitreous haemorrhage happens, it can cause sudden loss of vision in the worst situation, while the macula is damaged.

Exudates (EDs) appear as yellow or white structures with variable shapes in the retina. They are caused by leakage of lipid and proteins from damaged vessels and indicate increased blood vessel permeability. EDs can be further categorized as hard exudates (HEs), which have well-defined boundaries, and soft exudates (SEs), which have unclear boundaries. When exudates approach the macular region, they are associated with the risk of macular oedema. When exudates enter the macular centre, they are considered as sight-threatening lesions.

Neovascularizations (NVs) are caused by new blood vessel growth due to extensive lack of oxygen in retinal capillaries because of capillary closure. NVs appear as wheel-like networks and are usually located at the connection of vascular branches. They are weak and ruptured and

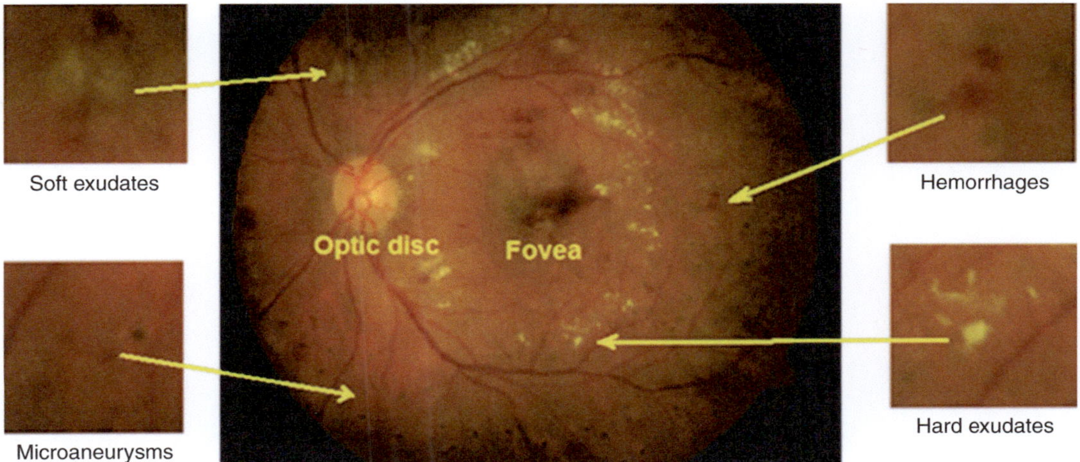

Fig. 2.1 Microaneurysms, haemorrhages and exudates in a colour fundus image

thereby able to cause loss of vision. For DR evaluation, commonly they can be grouped as NVs on the disc (NVD) and NVs elsewhere (NVE).

Besides the above-mentioned pathologies, cotton wool spots (CWS), venous beading (VB), pre-retinal haemorrhages and vitreous haemorrhages can be viewed in the different stages of DR progression. The emergence of neovascularizations, pre-retinal haemorrhages and vitreous haemorrhages can be considered a high-risk level of DR progression. Figure 2.1 illustrates the morphological and colorific characteristics of MAs, HMs and EDs in a colour fundus image.

2.3 DR Level Grading Standards

2.3.1 International Standard

Most of DR grading standards used in the DR screening programmes were based on the Early Treatment Diabetic Retinopathy Study (ETDRS) and Wisconsin Epidemiology Study of Diabetic Retinopathy publications [8].

In 2001, the American Academy of Ophthalmology (AAO) launched the Global Diabetic Retinopathy Project to promote the development of a common clinical severity scale for DR and DME [9]. Later, the International Clinical Diabetic Retinopathy and Diabetic Macular Oedema Disease Severity Scales were recommended by AAO for clinical practice. The International Severity Scales proposed five levels for grading of DR and 4 levels for grading DME based on the risk of DR progression. The classification standard allowed clinically important grades of retinopathy and allowed non-ophthalmologists, as optometrists and primary care physicians, attend DR screening. The international DR and DME severity scales are summarized in Table 2.1.

The AAO recommended, for Type I diabetes, first eye examination should be within 3–5 years, and the follow-up should be yearly after the first examination. For Type II diabetes, annual eye examination was recommended [10].

2.3.2 UK NSC Standard

The UK is another country conducting large-scale and community-based DR screening programmes. From 1990 to 2002, the UK adopted the European guidelines as DR grading system [11]. After 2003, the National Screening Committee (NSC), UK, introduced a new NSC grading system for digital photography-based DR screening [12]. Table 2.2 gives a summary about the levels of DR and DME in the grading system. The NSC grading standard

Table 2.1 International clinical DR disease and DME disease severity scales

Disease severity level	Description
DR	
No apparent retinopathy	No abnormalities
Mild NPDR	MAs only
Moderate NPDR	More than just MAs but less than severe NPDR
Severe NPDR	Any of the following: Extensive (>20) intraretinal HMs in each of 4 quadrants Definite VB in 2 more quadrants Prominent IRMA in 1 more quadrant No signs of PDR
PDR	One or more of the signs of: Neovascularizations Vitreous/pre-retinal HMs
DME	
DME apparently absent	No apparent retinal thickening or HEs in posterior pole
Mild DME	Retinal thickening and HEs in posterior pole but distant from the centre of the macula
Moderate DME	Retinal thickening or HEs approaching the centre of the macula but not involving the centre (500 µm radius of macular centre)
Severe DME	Retinal thickening or HEs involving the centre of the macula (500 µm radius of macular centre)

DR diabetic retinopathy, *DME* diabetic macular oedema, *MAs* microaneurysms, *HMs* haemorrhages, *HEs* hard exudates, *NPRD* non-proliferative diabetic retinopathy, *PDR* proliferative diabetic retinopathy, *VB* venous beading, *IRMA* intraretinal microvascular abnormalities

Table 2.2 UK NSC retinopathy grading standard

Retinopathy stage	Description
DR	
R0: none DR	No visible DR
R1: background DR	MAs, HMs, any exudates not with the definition of maculopathy
R2: pre-proliferative DR	VB, venous loop or reduplication, IRMA multiple deep, round or blot HMs
R3: proliferative	R3a: (active) NVD, NVE, pre-retinal or vitreous HM, pre-retinal fibrosis ± tractional retinal detachment R3s: (stable posttreatment) evidence of peripheral retinal laser treatment and stable retina from photographs at discharge from the Hospital Eye Service
DME	
M0: no visible DME	Absence of any M1 features
M1: DME	Exudates within 1 DD of macular centre, circinate or group of exudates with the macula retinal thickening with 1DD of the macular centre (if stereo available), any MA or HM within 1DD of the centre of the fovea only if associated with a best VA of <= 6/12 (if stereo unavailable)
Photocoagulation (P)	Evidence of focal/grid laser to macula, evidence of peripheral scatter laser
Unclassifiable (U)	Ungradable

UK NSC United Kingdom National Screening Committee, *DR* diabetic retinopathy, *DME* diabetic macular oedema, *MAs* microaneurysms, *HMs* haemorrhages, *VB* venous beading, *NVD* neovascularizations on the disc, *NVE* neovascularizations elsewhere, *VA* visual acuity, *IRMA* intraretinal microvascular abnormalities, DD disc diameter

was defined based on the ETDRS grading standard. The major difference from the international standard is that for proliferative DR, two levels, R3a (active) PDR and R3s (stable) PDR, are defined. An unclassifiable (ungradable) category was also added in the standard.

Another difference is the NSC standard that also defines grading pathway for DR screening. That is,

Table 2.3 A simplified version of the Wisconsin grading system for classifying DR (Australia)

Retinopathy stage	Description
DR	
Minimal NPDR	MA only
Mild NPDR	MA and one or more of: retinal HM, HE, CWS, but not meeting moderate NPDR
Moderate NPDR	HM/MA in at least one quadrant and one or more of: CWS, VB, IRMA
Severe NPDR	HM/Ma in all four quadrants, IRMA in one or more quadrants, VB in two or more quadrants
PDR	Any of: NVE, NVD, vitreous/pre-retinal haemorrhage
High-risk PDR	Any of: NVD > 1/4–1/3 disc area, or with vitreous/pre-retinal HM, or NVE > 1/2 disc area with vitreous/pre-retinal HM
Advanced PDR	High-risk PDR with traditional detachment involving the macula or vitreous haemorrhage obscuring ability to grade NVD and NVE
DME	
Macular oedema	Retinal thickening within two disc diameters of macular centre
Clinically significant macular oedema (CSME)	Retinal thickening within 500 μm of macular centre or HEs within 500 μm of macular centre with adjacent retinal thickening

DR Diabetic retinopathy, *MAs* microaneurysms, *HMs* haemorrhages, *VB* venous beading, *NPRD* non-proliferative diabetic retinopathy, *CWS* cotton wool spots, *NVD* neovascularizations on the disc, *NVE* neovascularizations elsewhere, *IRMA* intraretinal microvascular abnormalities, *PDR* proliferative diabetic retinopathy

firstly, all images are graded by a certificated primary grader. Then, the images will be graded by a certificated secondary grader who does not know the grading results from the primary grader. If the results from them are in disagreement, an arbitrator (retinal specialist) will grade the images and his decision will be used as the final ones.

2.3.3 Other Standards

The standards used by other countries as France, Australia, etc. are usually modified or simplified versions based on the ETDRS and Wisconsin grading systems. They are quite similar to the international standard but may have a minor difference.

Table 2.3 gives a standard recommended by the National Health and Medical Research Council, Australia.

2.4 DR Screening by Morphological Means

As above-mentioned standards, morphological means based on the shape and colour characteristics of DR pathologies are common methods used for DR screening. In a DR screening programme, several key factors should be considered. They are the eye examination method, role of medical staff, pathology identification method, DR grading standard and structure of screening network.

Conventional eye fundus examination methods, such as using indirect ophthalmoscope or slit lamp biomicroscopy on dilated eyes by ophthalmologists, have been proved effective for detecting retinopathy [13], but direct ophthalmoscopy by GPs for DR detection are less effective [14]. The limitation of the conventional methods is it is hard to offer a population-based DR screening. In the past decade, fundus photography, especially digital fundus imaging, has been proved be able to provide effective fundus examination as a role in DR screening [15–17]. Mydriatic fundus cameras on dilated eyes were used at the early stage. New non-mydriatic cameras without eye dilation have been commonly accepted now. Dilation is only provided for small pupil eyes if non-mydriatic imaging is not successful.

For DR screening, digital fundus camera has been proved its advantages [18], especially for providing excellent quality. The instant image acquisition with immediate image quality assessment can potentially reduce the technical failure rate for fundus imaging. And the digital images can make their storage and transmission much easy compared to the conventional eye fundus examinations. In the following, digital fundus imaging role in DR screening programme is emphasized.

For DR screening by using digital fundus camera, technically, a patient should undergo visual acuity measurement and fundus photography. 45° or 50° fundus cameras are commonly used for the fundus imaging in a darkened room. Several fundus images of each eye of the patient will be taken according to different DR screening standards. In the early stage of the DR screening programmes, most standards recommended five-field or three-field images (one is macula centred, one optic disc centred and one temporal to the macula) per eye [19, 20]. In the recent years, two-field imaging rule (macula centred and disc centred) has been accepted by most screening programmes [21].

Most screening standards recommend immediate image quality assessment after image acquisition. The French Association for the Study of Diabetes and Metabolic Diseases (ALFEDIAM) standard recommends five image quality levels: (1) excellent; (2) good definition of most retinal details; (3) definition limited, difficult to assess; (4) only gross detail visible; and (5) not gradable [19, 22]. UK NSC defines three image quality levels: (1) good, (2) adequate and (3) inadequate (ungradable). If the image quality is not satisfied, the imaging process can be repeated immediately.

Medical staff involving a DR screening programme can be simply categorized into two types. One is technician staff (or screeners) for taking fundus images by using digital fundus cameras. Through a training process, nurses, orthoptists, optometrists, etc. can fully undertake the role. Another kind of staff for DR screening is image grading staff, who undertake the task of reading fundus images, identifying pathologies and grading DR levels. Ophthalmologists are best persons for undertaking the DR grading task. However, because of lack of ophthalmologists, in a large-scale DR screening programme, other medical staff can be trained and undertake the image grading task. In UK NSC recommended screening system, the image grader's role and image grading pathway are set up. Certificated primary and secondary graders and arbitrators (eye specialists) play the grading roles in the defined image grading workflow. There were other studies which aimed at evaluating other clinical staff, as orthoptists, optometrists and GPs, for taking the grading task. For example, the California state-wide DR screening programme has included optometrists in its image reading system, who could review the patient's images as the same responsibility as ophthalmologists [23]. A recent study in Spain showed that GPs after adequate training could give high-level accuracy by using non-mydriatic photography for screening diabetes patients and refer the DR patients identified to ophthalmologists [24]. In Victoria, Australia, 45 orthoptists attended the DR image grading performance evaluation by using 36 digital images. A performance with the mean sensitivity of 86 % and specificity of 91 % for identifying abnormalities in the images was achieved [25]. Although the studies indicated that GPs, orthoptists, etc. could potentially act as graders in DR screening programmes after good training process, there are arguments that the ophthalmologist's role in DR image grading should not be reduced.

Image grading process usually includes identifying pathologies on colour fundus images and grading DR levels according to DR grading standards. Morphological features related to DR, as MAs, HMs, EDs, VB and NVs, are commonly identified by an image grader in an image reading phase. DR disease level can be graded according to the currently recommended DR grading standards, such as the international DR disease severity scales, UK NSC standard, etc. The screening results sent back to the GPs or screeners can include the severity of DR and advice for the referral/no referral of a patient for further examination or treatment or a follow-up examination in a defined interval. Basic criteria of a DR screening programme should target at providing sufficiently high sensitivity (true positive rate) and specificity (true negative rate). The high sensitivity can ensure that the patients with DR (as DR level above moderate NPDR or sight-threatening retinopathy) are not missed for referral and treatment. The high specificity, on the other hand, can ensure that the diabetes patients without reaching the level of referral are not referred. The UK NSC grading standard recommends 80 % sensitivity and specificity for DR screening programme [12].

Several solutions can be used to construct a DR screening network. One solution is to locate the fundus cameras in fixed community centres and let them be operated by trained health providers for image scanning. Another solution is to mount the fundus cameras on mobile vans for serving remote or rural areas. These two solutions also can be combined as a hybrid service model. A grading centre linked with the screening sites play an important role of image grading. Data transmission between the grading centre and screening sites with an efficient and secure mode becomes especially important for providing instant information feedback. With the universal application of the Internet in remote and rural areas, Internet-based patient information transmission can bridge the grading centre and screening sites efficiently. Especially, a specially designed tele-ophthalmology system will provide great convenience for a DR screening programme [26].

A tele-ophthalmology, which links a grading centre to its surrounding DR screening sites, can easily implement a DR screening workflow as the steps of: (1) the primary health providers scan patient's fundus images and transmit the images with the patient's other medical information and eye examination results to the grading centre [27]; (2) the eye grading experts (ophthalmologists or graders) read the images and grade the images according to a grading standard; (3) the grading results are transmitted back to the corresponding screening sites; and (4) the health providers inform the results to the patient and instruct for follow-up examination or treatment. In a tele-ophthalmology system, technically, the efficiency of the transmission of image is one of important factors. The original image size of the fundus image can be 1 Mbytes to several Mbytes depending on the resolution and dimensions of the image. Image compression method can be applied for the convenience of the image transmission through the Internet.

The telemedicine service model for DR screening programme can greatly save the ophthalmologists' or graders' time and let them provide efficient services to the patients living in a vast area. This service model has been implemented in some countries.

2.5 DR Screening Programmes in the World

DR screening programmes have been developed and practiced in some countries [28–30].

In France, the French National Health Authority recommended an annual examination of the eyes on diabetes patients without examination before or no mild retinopathy [31]. Two-field image scanning (macular centred and disc centred) was recommended. The French ALFEDIAM standard, which is quite similar to the international DR severity scales, was used for DR level classification [32].

In early 1990s, the DR screening programmes in France were practiced by using slit lamp biomicroscopy on dilated eyes. In France, the lack of qualified manpower (absence of optometrists) was a key problem for performing a wide DR screening, especially organizing an efficient and cost-effective DR screening programme [33]. In February 2002, the first DR screening centre by using telemedicine technique was set up in Paris. The orthoptists in the centre used a non-mydriatic fundus camera to take images for diabetes patients referred by GPs. The images were sent to a grading centre for DR grading. In 18 months, a total of 912 DR examinations were performed [19]. In June 2004, an ophthalmological diabetes telemedicine network "Ophdiat" was created in the Île-de-France area [34]. Seven hospitals, 11 primary healthcare centres and 2 prisons joined the DR screening programme. An average of seven ophthalmologists in the grading centre supported the DR grading task. From June 2004 to December 2009, 38,596 patients (in 51,741 examinations) were screened. Of the screening examinations, 13,726 (26.55 %) were referred to ophthalmologists. Through the screening programme, the telemedicine system has shown its reliability for providing one grading centre and multiple screening sites service model in a vast area.

An early DR screening programme in the USA is the Diabetes 2000 launched in 1990, which aimed at in 10 years eliminating preventable diabetes-related blindness in 2000 through early DR detection and treatment [35]. With the high prevalence of diabetes in the USA, the American Diabetes Association and AAO recommended annual eye examination for Type I and Type II diabetes patients. However, a high number of patients without access to annual DR screening existed in the USA [36]. It was estimated that half of diabetes patients attended the DR screening still through a traditional referral method by primary health providers. In 2011, a study showed establishing nationwide DR screening programmes was still a challenge [36] and new ideas to improve patient's compliance were needed. The role of telemedicine methods in DR screening programmes was discussed and practiced in the USA in the past decade. A telemedicine project in the University Pittsburgh Medical Center clinics graded 706 diabetes patients and demonstrated the success of the registration, imaging and grading workflow process. It has been shown the system could provide adequate screening and increase patient treatment compliance [37]. In California, a California HealthCare Foundation (CHCF)-supported teleretinal screening project EyePACS was set up in 2005, which used a web-based service model for patient DR image scanning (primary care providers at clinics) and image reading (ophthalmologists at reading centres) and grading result reporting. In 2005–2006, 3,562 cases were recorded. Later, the screening network was expanded to over 120 primary care sites [38]. In 2007, based on the pilot project, CHCF launched the Expanding Access to Diabetic Retinopathy Screening Initiative DR screening programme. At the end of 2010, over 53,000 cases had been screened [39].

The UK is one of the earliest countries starting DR screening programmes nationwide. Systematic DR screening by using digital fundus cameras in the UK has been practiced for 10 years. Before 2003, UK programmes used a descriptive DR grading system based on the Europe DR screening protocol. From 2003, the UK NSC recommended NSC grading system for UK national DR screening programme. Later, a new DR screening pathway based on the grading system, which used primary and secondary as two-level grading and an arbitrator as

arbitration in another level if necessary, was introduced [40]. In the UK, the grading standards among Scotland, Wales, England and North Ireland had minor difference, but the basic principles were the same. For example, in Scotland, single photography per eye was used, but in Wales and England, two-field images per eye were adopted. In 2002, Scotland started its first national DR screening programme. 150,000 diabetes patients participated in the annual eye examination [41]. Wales also started its national DR screening programme in 2002 [42, 43]. In 2006, 96 screening programmes started in England [44], which covered 350,000 people. The English national screening programme aimed at offering DR screening for all diabetes patients over the age of 12 years. In 2010–2011, the English screening programmes screened 1,790,000 patients among 2,260,000 patients offered for DR screening, reaching a nationwide uptake of 79 % [21]. Till the year 2012, England had set up more than 80 local programmes.

In Australia, the NHMRC recommended that the people with diabetes should attend annual or biennial eye examinations. The early Australian DR studies include Newcastle NSW study (1977–1988), Blue Mountain Eye Study (1992–1993), Melbourne Visual Impairment Project (1993–1994) [45] and Victorian township DR screening [46]. In 2003, a nationwide AusDiab study was performed in Australia. 11,247 adults were recruited for the DR screening. A simplified version of the Wisconsin grading system (Table 2.3) was adopted for DR level grading. 15.3 % of diabetes people had identified with DR [25].

In Bahrain [47], the first telemedicine-based DR screening programme was set up in 2003. From 2003 to 2009, six DR screening units were established for accumulatively 17,490 diabetes patients screened. Of the patients, 20.4 % were diagnosed with DR.

2.6 Validity of DR Screening Programmes

The validity of a screening programme can include the following factors: the quality of image acquisition, quality of image grading, efficiency of image grading result feedback and effectiveness of entire screening system.

In an Australian Kimberley DR screening programme in 2001, 680 images were selected and scored as excellent, adequate and inadequate for evaluating the acquired image quality. It has shown that over 90 % of photographs were excellent or adequate quality [48]. In the AusDiab study (2003) in Australia, the high degree of agreement between the first and second grading of DR ($k = 0.732$, unweighted) was achieved [25].

In the French telemedicine DR screening programme Ophdiat, a 5-year (2004–2009) experience on it summarized that telemedicine was a well DR screening method when our society was facing the prevalence of diabetes and the lack of ophthalmologist [32]. Through the telemedicine system, 93.9 % of the images could be graded on the same day. After introduction of the double regrading mechanism (each month, 5 % of patients in previous month are selected for regrading and may be judged by a senior ophthalmologist if there is disagreement) in 2008, the quality assurance of the image grading was further improved. In the 5-year Ophdiat project, the validity of screening programme has been shown. A total of around 73 % of all diabetes patients were graded as non-DR or mild DR. In 2008, 51.86 % of the patients attended annual examination. In the 5 years, the number of screening examinations increased steadily each year. These indicated the acceptance of the telemedicine DR screening by patients, ophthalmologists and GPs. From the 5-year experience, it concluded that both patients and ophthalmologist benefited from the Ophdiat system for efficiency and time saving [32].

In the UK, a study [49] reported the diabetes-related blindness decreased while the national DR screening programme had been implemented for 5 years in the Leeds metropolitan area. It showed the DR screening programmes with good control of systemic factors could greatly decrease the prevalence and incidence of DR, thereby reducing sight loss in diabetics. In Bristol and Weston (UK) DR screening programme, a prospective audit was performed on 213 image sets graded by six primary graders. An expert grader regraded all images. The audit result demonstrated a good interobserver agreement (better than the audit standard 80 % in all the categories). It meant the acceptable level of DR grading quality and accuracy from the primary graders [50]. The UK NSC grading standard recommends primary-secondary-arbitrator grading (universal and independent regrading) rule. A study was performed to evaluate the additional utility of universal regrading. 2,716 people with no DR graded by the primary graders were regraded by the secondary graders, and the disagreements were judged by the arbitrators. The universal regrading of normal images from the primary and secondary graders achieved 86.25 % concordance. It has shown the primary-secondary-arbitrator grading rule enhances the accuracy of DR detection [51]. In the NSC screening programmes, all graders were required to attend the national "Test and Training" set regularly. The NSC also made quality control standards and requested all screening programmes need to submit annual reports for data analysis and comparison. All these means helped to keep the quality assurance of the screening programmes.

In Bahrain's DR screening programme [47], a 1-year pilot project was initiated in one primary care unit for validating the telemedicine-based DR screening service model. After the effectiveness and feasibility were confirmed, a nationwide screening programme (six screening units) was established and moved forward. A similar manner of going from pilot project (2005–2006) to a complete DR screening programme (120 primary care sites) was used in California DR screening [38]. At the end of 2008, 34,100 cases had been screened.

The programmes indicated that for a network-based screening model, an initial investment in professional and material resources was needed. It could attract primary care providers to attend the screening programmes with minimal effort and resources but increase patients' compliance. The attendance of the primary care providers and the compliance of the patients could improve the validity of the screening programmes greatly.

2.7 Cost-Effectiveness of DR Screening Programmes

The cost associated with DR screening is of paramount importance for promoting screening programmes in vast regions, especially in remote and rural areas. In screening programmes, besides ophthalmologists, image graders and the type of equipments, the participation of GPs, primary health providers and nurses is also important to promise the cost-effectiveness. The service model of combining digital image cameras serving in fixed healthcare centres or in mobile vans with a telemedicine network has the potential to deliver cost-effective, accessible screening to urban and rural populations with diabetes.

In early 2000, a cost-effective simulation study on Type II diabetes patients showed that annual DR screening for Type II diabetics without previous DR detection might not provide cost-effectiveness. However, every third year screening for the diabetics with good glycemic control would be more cost-effective [52]. But UK's simulation model [53] (in 2002) on screening policy evaluation and relationship evaluation between cost-effectiveness with screening strategies gave a different result that there was not much cost-effectiveness while screening less than once a year. On the other hand, the simulation result indicated that systematic screening could provide the prevention of 50 % of the sight years lost caused by DR and showed more cost-effectiveness to screening outside an ophthalmic clinic. Now, an accepted view is that early detection and evidence-based treatment of DR can be cost-effective for preventing diabetes-related blindness [54, 55]. And systematic DR screening programme has been shown to be effective [56]. In the UK, nationwide DR screening has met its objectives that at least 80 % of eligible diabetes patients would be screened, recommended by the UK NSC.

The effectiveness of telemedicine system applied in DR screening programmes was discussed. A comparison on a tele-ophthalmology system using non-mydriatic camera with a clinic-based ophthalmoscopy examination by pupil dilation on PDR detection has shown that the tele-ophthalmology system was less costly and more effective. It is particularly cost-effective for preventing sight-threatening DR and vision loss [57]. A cost-effective study based on an Indian rural telemedicine DR screening project [58] reported that the 1-off (screening offered once) screening programme was cost-effective compared with no screening. Based on the regular intervals and sufficient screening coverage, screening every 2 years was also cost-effective.

An analysis report about California's EyePASC programme showed that telemedicine DR screening is a cost-effective approach. In 2007, the analysis indicated that each patient served in the system could contribute state cost savings with $2,500 over the patient's lifetime [23]. Considering some changes as increased cases, follow-up care, refined protocols, etc., the cost savings was updated to $768 per patient [39].

Conclusions

Screening for diabetic retinopathy involves retinal imaging of a population with a pre-defined illness, i.e. diabetes. The DR screening programme usually needs to consider the type of equipments, disease recognition methods, DR grading standards, screening service models and human resources. In the past decade, the DR screening programmes have shown that the digital fundus image-based DR screening method by morphological features of DR signs provides efficient early diagnosis. Combining digital imaging and telemedicine technology, the programmes can provide DR screening to the rural and remote areas, supported by the health providers and primary care providers. The telemedicine-based service model can also reduce the workload of ophthalmologists and cost of delivery of care due to complications and subsequent vision loss.

References

1. Juutilainen A, Lehto S, Rönnemaa T, Pyörälä K, Laakso M. Retinopathy predicts cardiovascular mortality in type 2 diabetic men and women. Diabetes Care. 2007;30:292–9.
2. Wong TY, Rosamond W, Chang PP, et al. Retinopathy and risk of congestive heart failure. JAMA. 2005; 293:63–9.
3. Edwards MS, Wilson DB, Craven TE, et al. Associations between retinal microvascular abnormalities and declining renal function in the elderly population: the Cardiovascular Health Study. Am J Kidney Dis. 2005;46:214–24.
4. http://www.who.int/mediacentre/factsheets/fs312/en/index.html. Online available: Sept 2012.
5. http://new.paho.org/hq/index.php?option=com_content&view=article&id=244&Itemid=1&lang=en&limitstart=1. Online available: Jan 2013.

6. Huang ES, Basu A, O'Grady M, Capretta JC. Projecting the future diabetes population size and related costs for the U.S. Diabetes Care. 2009;32(12):2225–9.

7. Silva PS, Cavallerano JD, Aiello LM, Aiello L. Telemedicine and diabetic retinopathy: moving beyond retinal screening. Arch Ophthalmol. 2011;129(2):236–42.

8. Early treatment of diabetic retinopathy study research group: grading diabetic retinopathy for stereoscopic colour fundus photographs an extension of the modified airlie house classification (report 10). Ophthalmology. 1991;98:786–806.

9. Wilkinson CP, Ferris FL, Klein RE, Lee PP, Agardh CD, Davis M, Dills D, Kampik A, Pararajasegaram R, Verdaguer JT. Proposed international clinical diabetic retinopathy and diabetic macular oedema disease severity scales. Ophthalmology. 2003;10(9):1677–82.

10. American Academy of Ophthalmology Retina Panel, Preferred Practice Pattern – Diabetic Retinopathy. Am Acad Ophthalmol. 2008. http://one.aao.org/CE/PracticeGuidelines/PPP.aspx. Online available: Aug 2013.

11. Retinopathy Working Party. A protocol for screening for diabetic retinopathy in Europe. Diabet Med. 1991;8:263–7.

12. UK National Screening Committee, Essential Elements in Developing a Diabetic Retinopathy Screening Programme. http://diabeticeye.screening.nhs.uk/. Online available: Aug 2013.

13. Owens DR, Dolben J, Young S, Ryder REJ, Jones IR, Vora J, et al. Screening for diabetic retinopathy (symposium). Diabet Med. 1991;8:S4–10.

14. Hulme SA, Tin-U A, Hardy KJ, Joyce PW. Evaluation of a district-wide screening programme for diabetic retinopathy utilizing trained optometrists using slit-lamp and Volk lenses. Diabetes UK, Diabet Med. 2002;19:741–5.

15. Squirrell DM, Talbot JF. Screening for diabetic retinopathy. J R Soc Med. 2003;96(6):273–6.

16. Massin P, Erginay A, Ben Mehidi A, et al. Evaluation of a new nonmydriatic digital camera for detection of diabetic retinopathy. Diabet Med. 2003;20:635–41.

17. Lin DY, Blumenkranz MS, Brothers RJ, Grosvenor DM. The Digital Diabetic Screening Group, The sensitivity and specificity of single-field nonmydriatic monochromatic digital fundus photography with remote image interpretation for diabetic retinopathy screening: a comparison with ophthalmoscopy and standardized mydriatic color photography. Am J Ophthalmol. 2002;134(2):204–13.

18. Rudnisky CJ, Hinz BJ, Tennant MT, et al. High resolution stereoscopic digital fundus photography versus contact lens biomicroscopy for the detection of clinically significant macular oedema. Ophthalmology. 2002;109:267–74.

19. Massin P, Aubert JP, Erginay A, Bourovitch JC, BenMehidi A, Audran G, Bernit B, Jamet M, Collet C, Laloi-Michelin M, Guillausseau PJ, Gaudric A, Marre M. Screening for diabetic retinopathy: the first telemedical approach in a primary care setting in France. Diabetes Metab. 2004;30(5):451–7.

20. Creuzot-Garcher C, Malvitte L, Sicard AC, Guillaubey A, Charles A, Beiss JN, Bron A. How to improve screening for diabetic retinopathy: the Burgundy experience. Diabetes Metab. 2010;36(2):114–9.

21. Peto T, Tadros C. Screening for diabetic retinopathy and diabetic macular oedema in the United Kingdom. Curr Diab Rep. 2012;12:338–45.

22. Massin P, Angioi-Duprez K, Bacin F, et al. Recommandations de l'ALFEDIAM pour le dépistage et la surveillance de la rétinopathie diabétique. Diabetes Metab. 1996;22:203–9.

23. Newman M. Fiscal impact of AB 175: analysis of the cost effectiveness of store and forward teleophthalmology: Blue Sky Consulting Group, 2009. http://www.chcf.org. Online available: Aug 2013.

24. Andonegui J, Zurutuza A, Arcelus MPD, Serrano L, Eguzkiza A, Auzmendi M, Gaminde I, Aliseda D. Diabetic retinopathy screening with non-mydriatic retinography by general practitioners: 2-year results. Prim Care Diabetes. 2012;6:201–5.

25. Georgievski Z, Koklanis K, Fenton A, KouKouras I. Victorian orthoptists' performance in the photo evaluation of diabetic retinopathy. Clin Experiment Opthalmol. 2007;35:733–8.

26. Lee P, Durham NC. Telemedicine, opportunities and challenges for the remote care of diabetic retinopathy. Arch Ophthalmol. 1999;117:1639–40.

27. Massin P, Aubert JP, Eschwege E, Erginay A, Bourovitch JC, BenMehidi A, Nougarède M, Bouéee S, Fagnani F, Tcherny MS, Jamet M, Bouhassira M, Marre M. Evaluation of a screening program for diabetic retinopathy in a primary care setting Dodia (Dépistage ophtalmologique du diabète) study. Diabetes Metab. 2005;31(2):153–62.

28. Rubino A, Rousculp MD, Davis K, Wang J, Girach A. Diagnosed diabetic retinopathy in France, Italy, Spain, and the United Kingdom. Prim Care Diabetes. 2007;1(2):75–80.

29. Kilstad HN, Sjølie AK, Gøransson L, Hapnes R, Henschien HJ, Alsbirk KE, Fossen K, Bertelsen G, Holstad G, Bergrem H. Prevalence of diabetic retinopathy in Norway: report from a screening study. Acta Ophthalmol. 2012;90:609–12.

30. Hansen AB, Andersen MVN. Screening for diabetic retinopathy in Denmark: the current status. Acta Ophthalmol Scand. 2004;82(6):673–8.

31. Massin P, Angioi-Duprez K, Bacin F, et al. Recommendations of the ALFEDIAM (French Association for the Study of Diabetes and Metabolic Diseases) for the screening and surveillance of diabetic retinopathy. J Fr Ophtalmol. 1997;20:302–10.

32. Schulze-Döbold C, Erginay A, Robert N, Chabouis A, Massin P. Ophdiat(®): five-year experience of a telemedical screening programme for diabetic retinopathy in Paris and the surrounding area. Diabetes Metab. 2012;38(5):450.

33. Deb N, Thuret G, Estour B, Massin P, Gain P. Screening for diabetic retinopathy in France. Diabetes Metab. 2004;30:140–5.

34. Massin P, Chabouis A, Erginay A, Viens-Bitker C, Lecleire-Collet A, Meas T, et al. OPHDIAT: a telemedical

network screening system for diabetic retinopathy in the Île-de-France. Diabetes Metab. 2008;34:227–34.

35. Hazin R, Colyer M, Lum F, Barazi MK. Revisiting Diabetes 2000: challenges in establishing nationwide diabetic retinopathy prevention programs. Am J Ophthalmol. 2011;152:723–9.

36. Hazin R, Barazi MK, Summerfield M. Challenges to establishing nationwide diabetic retinopathy screening programs. Curr Opin Ophthalmol. 2011;22(3):174–9.

37. Wilson RR, Silowash R, Anthony L, Cecil RA, Eller A. Telemedicine process used to implement an effective and functional screening program for diabetic retinopathy. J Diabetes Sci Technol. 2008;2(5):785–91.

38. Cuadros J, Bresnick G. EyePACS: an adaptable telemedicine system for diabetic retinopathy screening. J Diabetes Sci Technol. 2009;3(3):509–16.

39. Quade R, Aulakh V. Chapter 15. Economics of screening for diabetic retinopathy using telemedicine in California's safety net. Digital teleretinal screening. Springer Heidelberg New York Dordrecht, London. 2012. ISBN 9783642258091.

40. Misra A, Bachmann MO, Greenwood RH, Jenkins C, Shaw A, Barakat O, Flatman M, Jones CD. Trends in yield and effects of screening intervals during 17 years of a large UK community-based diabetic retinopathy screening programme. Diabet Med. 2009;26:1040–7.

41. Christie B. Scotland to start screening programme for diabetic retinopathy. BMJ. 2002;324(7342):871.

42. Welsh Assembly Government. National Service Framework for Diabetes in Wales – Delivery strategy. 2003. http://www.wales.nhs.uk/documents/DiabetesNSF_eng. pdf. Online available: Aug 2013.

43. Yeo ST, Edwards RT, Luzio SD, Charles JM, Thomas RL, Peters JM, Owens DR. Diabetic retinopathy screening: perspectives of people with diabetes, screening intervals and costs of attending screening. Diabet Med. 2012;29:878–85.

44. Scanlon PH. The English national screening programme for sight-threatening diabetic retinopathy. J Med Screen. 2008;15(1):1–4.

45. McCarty CA, Lloyd-Smith CW, Lee SE, Livingston PM, Stanislavsky YL, Taylor HR. Use of eye care services by people with diabetes: the Melbourne Visual Impairment Project. Br J Ophthalmol. 1998;82(4):410–4.

46. Harper AC, Livingstone PM, Wood C, et al. Screening for diabetic retinopathy using a non-mydriatic retinal camera in rural Victoria. Aust N Z J Ophthalmol. 1998;26:117–21.

47. Alawi EA, Ahmed AA. Screening for diabetic retinopathy: the first telemedicine approach in a primary care setting in Bahrain. Middle East Afr J Ophthalmol. 2012;19(3):295–8.

48. Mak DB, Plant AJ, McAllister I. Screening for diabetic retinopathy in remote Australia: a program description and evaluation of a developed model. Aust J Rural Health. 2003;11:224–30.

49. Arora S, Kolb S, Goyder E, McKibbin MM. Trends in the incidence of visual impairment resulting from diabetic retinopathy in the Leeds metropolitan area. Diabet Med. 2012;29(7):e112–6.

50. Patra S, Gomm EMW, Macipe M, Bailey C. Interobserver agreement between primary graders and an expert grader in the Bristol and Weston diabetic retinopathy screening programme: a quality assurance audit. Diabet Med. 2009;26:820–3.

51. Manjunatha RS, Manjunatha NP, Baskar V, Headon MP, Singh BM, Viswanath AK. Quality assurance in the diabetic retinopathy screening programme: evaluating the benefit of universal regrading of the normal primary grade. Diabet Med. 2012;29(2):287–8.

52. Vijan S, Hofer TP, Hayward RA. Cost utility of screening intervals for diabetic retinopathy in patients with type 2 diabetes mellitus. JAMA. 2000;283:889–96.

53. Davies R, Roderick P, Canning C, Brailsford S. The evaluation of screening policies for diabetic retinopathy using simulation. Diabet Med. 2002;19:762–70.

54. Tung T, Shih H, Chen S, Chou P, Liu C, Liu J. Economic evaluation of screening for diabetic retinopathy among Chinese type 2 diabetics: a community-based study in Kinmen, Taiwan. J Epidemiol. 2008;18(5):225–33.

55. Polak BC, Crijns H, Casparie AF, Niessen LW. Cost-effectiveness of glycaemic control and ophthalmological care in diabetic retinopathy. Health Policy. 2003;64:89–97.

56. Jones S, Edwards RT. Diabetic retinopathy screening: a systematic review of the economic evidence. Diabet Med. 2009;27:249–56.

57. Whited JD, Datta SK, Aiello LM, et al. A modeled economic analysis of a digital tele-ophthalmology system as used by three federal health care agencies for detecting proliferative diabetic retinopathy. Telemed J E Health. 2005;11(6):641–51.

58. Rachapelle S, Legood RA, Alavi Y, Lindfield R, Sharma T, Kuper H, Polack S. The cost–utility of telemedicine to screen for diabetic retinopathy in India. Ophthalmology. 2013;120(3):566–73.

Multimodal Screening of Glaucoma Improves Sensitivity and Specificity

Folkert K. Horn and Werner Adler

Contents

F.K. Horn, PhD (✉)
Department of Ophthalmology, University
Eye Hospital, Friedrich-Alexander University
Erlangen-Nürnberg, Erlangen, Germany

Universitäts-Augenklinik, Schwabachanlage 6,
D-91054 Erlangen, Germany

Department of Ophthalmology, University Medical
Center Erlangen, Erlangen, Germany
e-mail: folkert.horn@uk-erlangen.de

W. Adler, PhD
Department of Medical Informatics, Biometry
and Epidemiology, Friedrich-Alexander University
Erlangen-Nürnberg, Erlangen D-91054 Germany
e-mail: werner.adler@fau.de

3.1   Introduction

Early glaucoma detection is crucial for prognosis of the disease and treatment to prevent ongoing damage of the visual field. Therefore, different setups to uncover glaucomatous defects at an early stage have been suggested. Diagnosis of glaucoma is very closely associated with morphologic changes in the optic nerve head and thus one screening parameter might consider the morphology of the optic disc. A further screening measurement should deliver information about the functional integrity of the visual system. In recent years, several sensory tests as well as morphological techniques have been developed to detect early glaucomatous defects, and the usefulness of combined evaluation of these data has been documented [1–7]. In the present evaluation, two methods have been applied in the same cohort of patients utilizing two current techniques: analysis of the optic nerve head with a scanning laser device (HRT) and visual field testing with the frequency doubling technology (FDT). The morphology of the optic nerve head can be mapped using the Heidelberg Retina Tomograph (HRT), which generates topographic images of the optic nerve head utilizing a confocal scanning diode laser. It has been shown that these topographic images can be used to detect glaucomatous optic nerve heads [8–11] at an early stage in some patients, partially even in eyes without measurable standard perimetric field loss at the time of measurement [12, 13].

G. Michelson (ed.), *Teleophthalmology in Preventive Medicine*,
DOI 10.1007/978-3-662-44975-2_3, © Springer-Verlag Berlin Heidelberg 2015

In FDT perimetry, localized defects in the visual field, as well as malfunctions of temporal transfer properties, may contribute to the results. In the past, the utility of this method has been shown for full-threshold strategies similar to those used with automated standard perimeters as well as for screening procedures [14–16]. Both methods might also be incorporated in a screening setup as the procedures are fast and outcomes are available for further processing directly after assessment.

Our aim was to develop classification rules for combined analysis of data from HRT measurements and FDT perimetry in preperimetric and perimetric glaucoma eyes using a machine-learning method. The difference between the FDT and the HRT was pointed out by the examination of preperimetric and perimetric glaucomas. In preperimetric glaucoma groups, patients revealed glaucomatous optic disc atrophy (defined by loss of neuroretinal rim [17]) and normal visual field testing with white-on-white perimetry. "Perimetric" patients showed glaucomatous optic disc atrophy and definite visual field defects. With the HRT performing well in the first subgroup and the FDT performing well in the second, we could examine the benefit of combining both instruments in a single classifier. In this study a random forest analysis [18] is used to build a predictive model. To obtain an estimation of the classifier's performance and to avoid unrealistically optimistic classification rates, we used independent populations for training and testing. Additional aim of our study was to demonstrate the application of a machine-learning method in the World Wide Web. Therefore, the classifier trained on the present learning cohort is provided via the Internet. This should allow scientists and user of the devices to calculate the probability of own observations to be normal or glaucoma.

3.2 Methods

3.2.1 Procedures

The study includes two completely separate and independent populations each containing controls, preperimetric and perimetric glaucoma patients: one population for the determination of machine-learning classifiers. This population contained participants of the Erlangen glaucoma registry [19]. The second population included patients who were recruited from the Erlangen University Eye Hospital. None of the participants was in both of the present populations. Numbers of subjects and demographic characteristics in every group are summarized in Table 3.1. All controls and patients were thoroughly examined by slit-lamp inspection, tonometry, funduscopy, gonioscopy, perimetry, and papillometry. The papillometric evaluations of the subjects and patients were based on color stereo photographs. Criteria for the diagnosis of glaucoma were glaucomatous changes of the optic nerve head including an unusually small neuroretinal rim area in relation to the optic disc size and cup-to-disc ratios being higher vertically compared to horizontal [17, 20]. All optic disc photographs were inspected and classified by at least three glaucoma specialists in a masked fashion so that the examiners were unaware of the diagnosis, intra-

Table 3.1 Demographic characteristics for all subgroups

	Definition		Training data set		Test data set	
	Visual field		"Erlangen Glaucoma Registry"		Outpatient department of "Erlangen University Eye Hospital"	
Group	Losses (octopus)	Evaluation of optic disc photographs	Number	Age [years]	Number	Age [years]
Control	No	Normal	161	53.8 ± 10.2	93	55.6 ± 6.0
Preperimetric Glaucoma	No	Glaucomatous Optic disc	102	55.8 ± 9.7	47	56.5 ± 6.3
Perimetric Glaucoma	Yes	Glaucomatous Optic disc	130	55.6 ± 8.9	55	58.3 ± 5.2

ocular pressure, and visual field data. All subjects underwent visual field testing with standard white-on-white perimetry with a computerized static projection perimeter (Octopus 500 or 101, program G1). Subjects with more than 12 % false-positive or false-negative responses in standard perimetry were not included. All individuals included in the study had an open anterior chamber angle, clear optic media, a visual acuity of 20/40 or better, and a myopic refractive error not exceeding −8 diopters. All individual morphologic and sensory data were obtained within a 48 h period. Range of age was 34–71 years in the training cohort and 45–65 years in the present test population. The registered study (www.clinicaltrials.gov, NCT00494923) was approved by the Institutional Review Board and followed the tenets of the declaration of Helsinki for research involving human subjects. Informed consent was obtained from all participants.

3.2.2 Subjects and Patient

Controls: The reference sample included randomly selected eyes of healthy control subjects from the Erlangen glaucoma registry. The control subjects of the test sample were healthy chaperons of patients or patients of the University Eye Hospital who had treatment (e.g., cataract surgery, no glaucoma) in the second eye. In all control eyes of this study, slit-lamp inspection, perimetry, tonometry, funduscopy, and papillometry were normal.

"Preperimetric" glaucoma patients: In the "preperimetric" glaucoma groups, patients showed glaucomatous abnormalities of the optic disc. Computerized visual field examinations with white-on-white perimetry were normal. The results of measurements on one randomly selected eye of each patient were used in the study.

"Perimetric" glaucoma patients: All patients of these groups had glaucomatous optic disc damage and pathological cumulative perimetric defect curves, i.e., local and/or diffuse visual field loss in white-on-white perimetry. Visual field losses of conventional white-on-white perimetry (Octopus standard index; perimetric mean defect) were

6.9 ± 5.3 dB in the training and 7.1 ± 4.2 dB in the test population. In both perimetric glaucoma groups, one eye of each patient was selected for the assessment of validity; this was always the eye with more advanced perimetric loss.

3.2.3 Screening with FDT Perimetry

The FDT perimeter (Zeiss Humphrey Systems) tests local contrast sensitivity in the central visual field. The technique has been described as a helpful test for diagnosing glaucoma [14, 21–23]. The device uses the frequency doubling phenomenon: if a low-spatial-frequency sine-wave grating pattern (0.25c/deg) is alternated with a temporal high-frequency (25 Hz) counter-phase flicker, the spatial frequency seems to be double that of the actual spatial frequency. In the present FDT test strategies (C-20-5 or N-30-5), this stimulus is presented in one of 17 target locations on a random basis. In the software version N-30-5 of the FDT perimeter, two more test locations are studied in a separate step of the test procedure. These additional tests are not considered in the present evaluation. The stimulus presentation consists of four targets per quadrant approximately 10° in diameter and one central 5° radius target. Each stimulus was presented maximally 0.4 s on a screen with a constant time-averaged luminance (100 cd/m²). The interstimulus interval was variable in order to reduce anticipation and rhythmic responses by the patient. Two types of catch trials were generated to attract the subject's attention and to obtain an impression of the goodness of the fixation. A 1-degree catch trial pattern at the location of the optic disc and a zero-contrast false-positive catch trial were randomly presented three times each. Subjects with more than one of the six catch trials positive were not included in this study, but the test was repeated. Before testing with the FDT perimeter, the subjects were shown a card with examples of the gratings to make them familiar with the test location and the stripe pattern. During the test, all other light sources, except the control monitors, were switched off in the examination room and a learning procedure was run. Patients were instructed to fixate the square tar-

Table 3.2 Results of the subjects in all subgroups of the study: the overall defect score in FDT perimetry and measures of the optic disc (total size of the optic disc and the area of the neuroretinal rim)

	Training data set				Test data set			
Group	n	Disc size [mm^2]	Rim area [mm^2]	FDT score	n	Disc size [mm^2]	Rim area [mm^2]	FDT score
Control	161	2.25±0.51	1.59±0.29	0.6±1.40	93	2.29±0.53	1.57±0.3	0.45±1.1
Preperimetric Glaucoma	102	2.45±0.53	1.34±0.31	4.2±7.1	47	2.46±0.46	1.39±0.27	1.7±2.9
Perimetric Glaucoma	130	2.37±0.48	1.02±0.32	28.3±18.3	55	2.36±0.55	1.04±0.36	28.7±20.1

FDT frequency doubling technique

get in the middle of the FDT screen and to press a response button if the flickering stripe pattern appeared anywhere on the monitor. Both eyes of the subjects were examined using the screening program C-20-5 with a 2 min rest period between the first (right) and second (left) eye [24]. This procedure presents stimuli with a contrast that 95 % of the normal population of the corresponding age group is able to detect. If the stimulus was detected, it was assumed that contrast sensitivity is within normal limits, and no further testing was performed at that location. If the initial stimulus was missed, the same stimulus was presented at that location a second time. If it was missed again, the instrument presented a stimulus with a contrast detectable by 98 % of the normal population, and if this was missed, a stimulus with a contrast detectable by 99 % of the normative subjects was presented. This strategy allows generating a score ranging from zero (i.e., first presentation seen) to four (i.e., 99 % level not seen) for all test locations. Considering all fields, the score ranges from 0 to 68 and from 0 to 16 in single quadrants [25]. The total FDT score is given for all groups in Table 3.2.

3.2.4 Heidelberg Retina Tomograph (HRT)

The Heidelberg Retina Tomograph (HRT I or HRT III for the reference sample, HRT II for the test sample), which generates stereometric measurements of the optic nerve head, was used to examine the morphology of the optic nerve head. A series of confocal images is obtained at consecutive focal planes and converted by the HRT software into a single tomographic image. To allow inclusion of results from the earlier HRT machines, we reanalyzed all data using the HRT III software which is backward compatible to earlier versions. To analyze the morphology of the optic nerve head, we included parameters derived from HRT images both globally and within six sectors as pre-given by the HRT. Several more newly given parameter of the HRT (e.g., steepness of the rim, glaucoma probability index) had been omitted in the present calculation because these parameter were not available in all data sets. The sector-related and global standard HRT parameters characterize volume and area of the neuroretinal rim, steepness of the cup (third moment), mean and peak height of the contour line, its height variation, the maximum depth of the cup, the papilla radius, and further volume and surface measures. The analysis includes linear discriminant formulas [26] (FSM-LDF, RB-LDF) and a score considering MRA classification in six sectors ranging from 0 to 12. Results in normal subjects and different glaucoma groups have been published earlier [27, 28]. In addition we tested a "corrected rim area" taking into account the dependency of the rim areas on the size of the optic disc [11, 29, 30] and the age of the subject similar to what was suggested earlier (Moorfields regression analysis). Instead of the originally published equation [11] which is recommended for subjects with optic discs between 1.2 and 2.8 mm^2, we used a slightly modified formula as in our subjects the range of the optic disc size was larger. For calculation of the present correction formula of the rim areas, we used all the data of 480

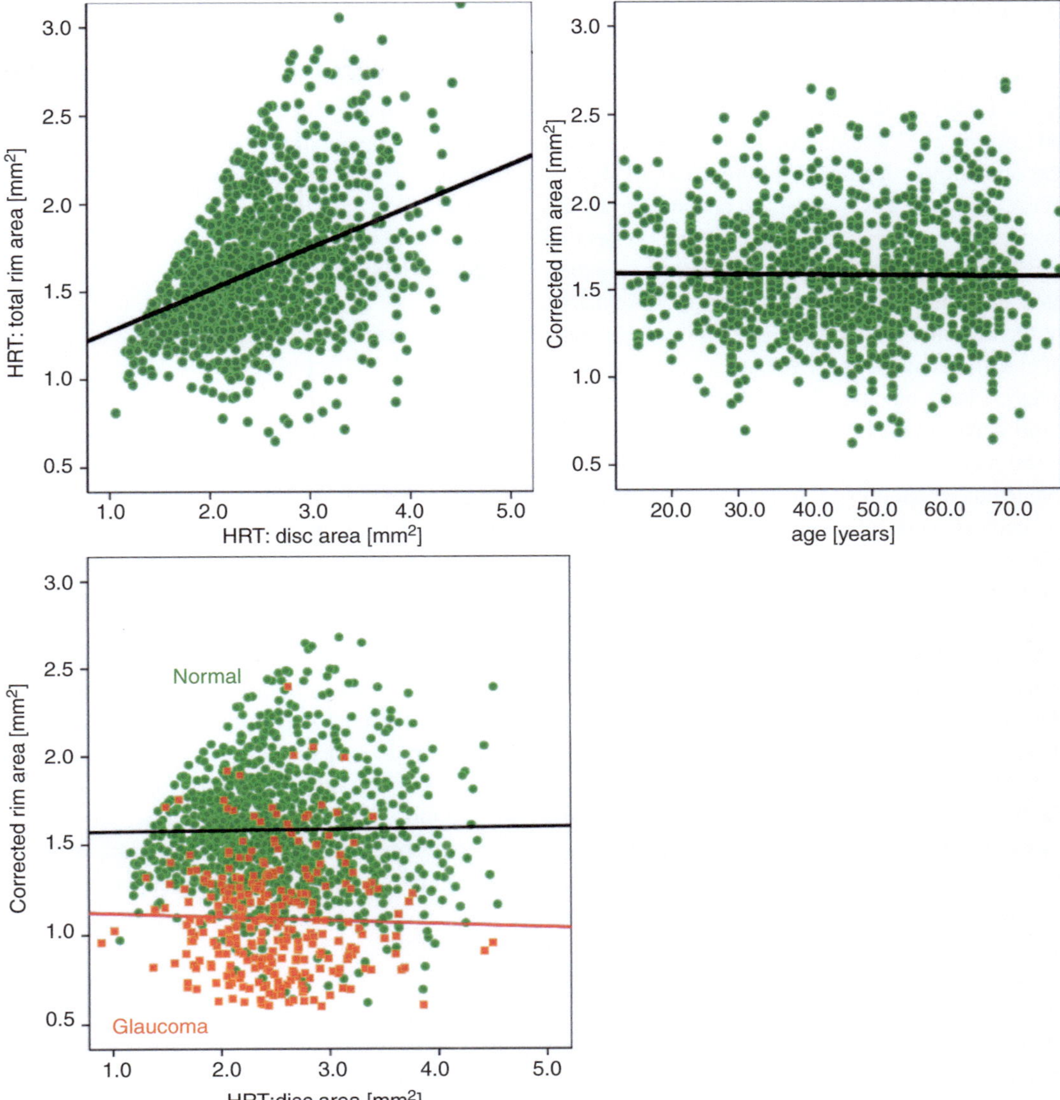

Fig. 3.1 Rim area versus disc area for all control eyes of the Erlangen glaucoma registry (*upper, left*). *Upper right* and *lower plot: Middle, right*: the same population after correction for disc size and age using the regression equation ("corrected rim area"=a*rim area/(b*disc area−c*age)). A group of glaucoma patients (*red symbols*) is included in the right lower figure to visualize the usefulness of this method in patients. A subgroup (see present inclusion criteria) of this normals and patients serves as learning cohort. *HRT* Heidelberg Retina Tomograph

healthy control eyes available from the Erlangen glaucoma registry. In this control group, the equation used for the correction of the rim size was: rim area = 1.2424 + 0.206 (disc area) − 0.003 (age). Figure 3.1 shows the relationship between neuroretinal rim and disc area for all control subjects of the Erlangen glaucoma registry using the present correction of the rim area. For the calculations in the present analysis, the patients with optic disc areas smaller than 1.3 mm² and larger than 3.7 mm² were not included because such values were not in all groups.

3.2.5 Automated Classification

In total, 112 variables were used to train the random forest classifier. We used four FDT sector scores, one overall FDT score, four sector differences and the upper/lower hemifield difference as FDT variables, and 102 HRT variables obtained from the instrument for the combined classifier. A second classifier using the HRT variables only was generated to compare this method with built-in LDFs of the machine. Random forest [18] is an ensemble of classification trees [31, 32], i.e., a large number of trees are built, where each tree uses a different bootstrap sample of the learning data. The decision of the forest then is obtained by majority voting. The special feature of a random forest is the way the trees are created. At every split point of the tree, the features, which are used to describe the split point, are drawn from a randomly selected subset of all variables. In earlier studies it could be shown that the random forest performs comparable or even better than other machine-learning methods [33]. Performance speed is a further advantage of the method. It can be installed on any personal computer. The analysis of our data was treated as a three-class problem, with the normal, preperimetric, and perimetric glaucoma classes. A random forest consisting of 500 trees was built using the learning population. The observations of the test data then were classified using this method. In the analysis, receiver operating characteristic (ROC) curves were used to describe the diagnostic performance of the discriminant analysis models of the HRT and the newly generated glaucoma classifiers. To be able to do an ROC analysis, we performed separate analyses for the preperimetric and the perimetric subgroups.

Using random forests, a proximity matrix between observations is generated, i.e., the similarity between the observations is computed. The proximity between observations is increased if they end up in the same leaf of one tree. This is done for all trees of the forest and a proximity matrix between all observations is created. This matrix can be visualized by multidimensional scaling (MDS) plots [34]. Multidimensional scaling [35] performs a dimension reduction, which facilitates the plotting of the proximity of the observations in two dimensions. Classification rules were examined in the free data analysis environment R (version

2.9.1, www.r-project.org). We additionally introduced an Internet browser tool for application of our trained classifier for telemedicine, diagnosis, and research via the World Wide Web. This tool utilized an open-source R package (RPAD), a data analysis software for shared application.

3.3 Results

3.3.1 Learning Glaucoma Classification

As we wanted to use the benefit from the characteristic strengths of HRT and FDT, the present classification system was trained with all available parameters from both devices. In order to avoid overoptimistic classification performance, we used a learning cohort that is independent from the test population. This learning data set includes 232 glaucoma patients and 161 control subjects. Figure 3.2 shows a comparison of the performance of the best twenty out of the 112 single variables. These variables were ranked by importance of the variables in the constructed trees for the total learning cohort. This construction takes into account how performance changes when a variable is part of the randomly selected input set compared to

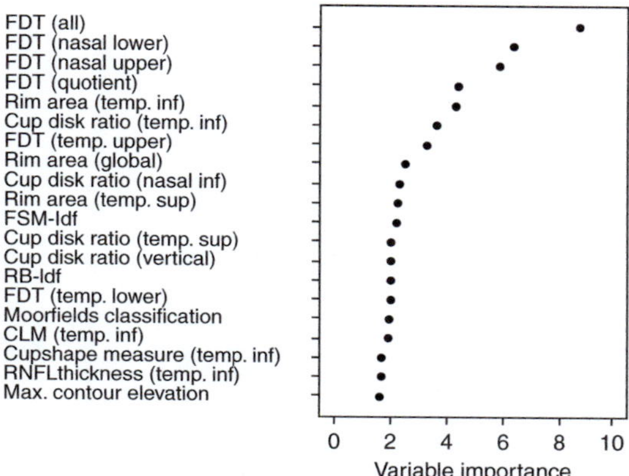

Fig. 3.2 Twenty most important variables of both diagnostic instruments ranked by the prediction accuracy for giving the correct classification. The variable importance measure was determined by the random forest method using the data of the learning data set. *FSM-ldf, RB-ldf* built-in classifiers using linear discriminant functions, *CLM* contour line modulation, *RNFL* retinal nerve fiber layer, *temp* temporal, *inf* inferior, *sup* superior, *FDT* frequency doubling technology

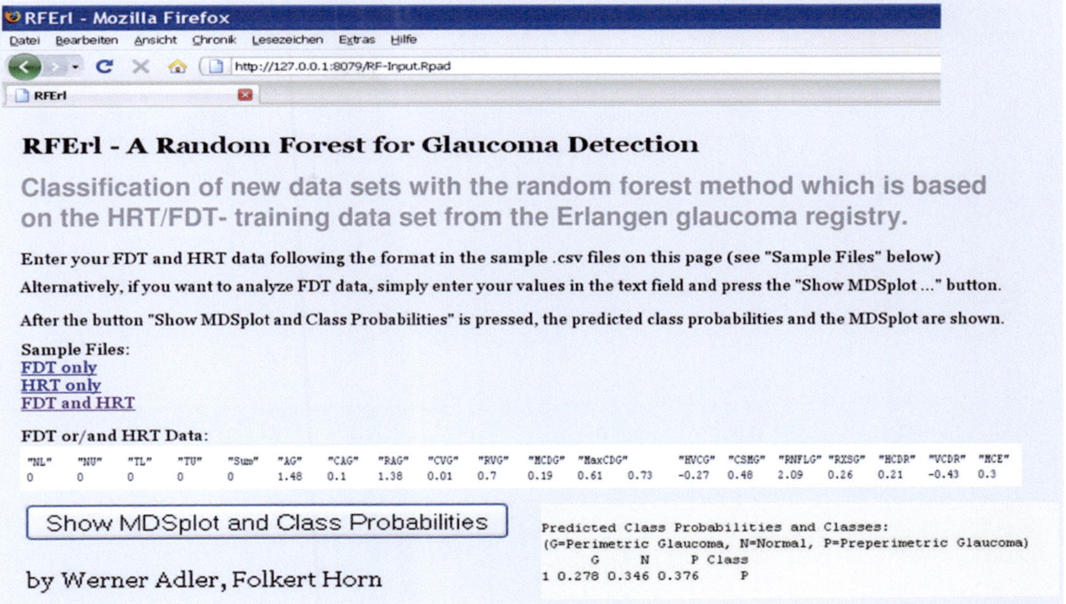

"NL"	"NU"	"TL"	"TU"	"Sum"	"AG"	"CAG"	"RAG"	"CVG"	"RVG"	"MCDG"	"MaxCDG"		"HVCG"	"CSMG"	"RNFLG"	"RXSG"	"HCDR"	"VCDR"	"MCE"
0	0	0	0	0	1.48	0.1	1.38	0.01	0.7	0.19	0.61	0.73	-0.27	0.48	2.09	0.26	0.21	-0.43	0.3

Fig. 3.3 An Internet browser tool was developed for the classification of new data sets from FDT perimetry and/or HRT. *HRT* Heidelberg Retina Tomograph, *FDT* frequency doubling technology. This platform includes all information of our learning cohort and can be easily installed on every computer. It generates the predicted class probability (*yellow field*) and an MDS (multidimensional scaling) plot for new data

performance when a variable is left out. This estimation of the variable importance in the total trained forest does not necessarily reflect the discriminative power of single variables to separate normals and a specific patient group. However, this graph gives an impression of the high importance of the score values and the hemifield difference of the FDT and the importance of LDF values, cup disc area ratios, and rim areas of the HRT. As the machine-learning classification system has been populated with data from well-known and clearly classified patients and controls, every new patient can be classified immediately after the measurement session. Figure 3.3 shows an Internet browser-based application software that can be used to classify new subjects based on the data from the present learning cohort. The results of HRT, FDT, or both can be loaded via csv file or imported directly by "copy and paste" using our platform. After data import the predicted class probability and the MDS plot are generated as can be seen in Fig. 3.4. This example (used in Fig. 3.3) indicates a predicted probability of 37.6 % to be preperimetric OAG and shows the estimated

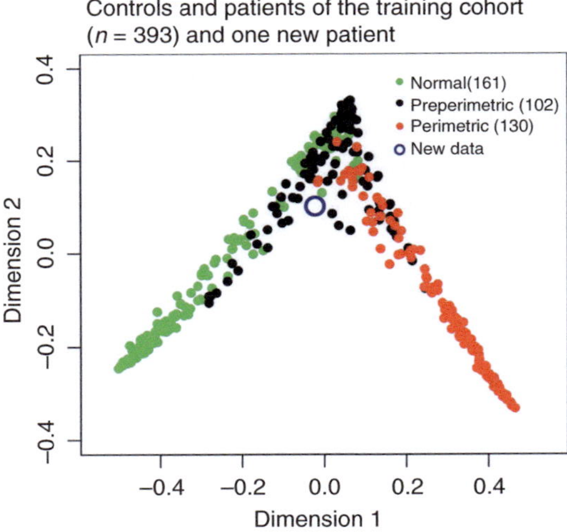

Fig. 3.4 Graphical presentation of our classification system in normals and patients of the training cohort. The shown multidimensional scaling plot is a projection of the total data to a two-dimensional surface. The colors indicate the real class of the subjects from the learning data set (controls: *green*, perimetric: *red*, preperimetric: *black*). The *blue ring* indicates class probability of a new patient as evaluated with the present classification tool (see Fig. 3.3)

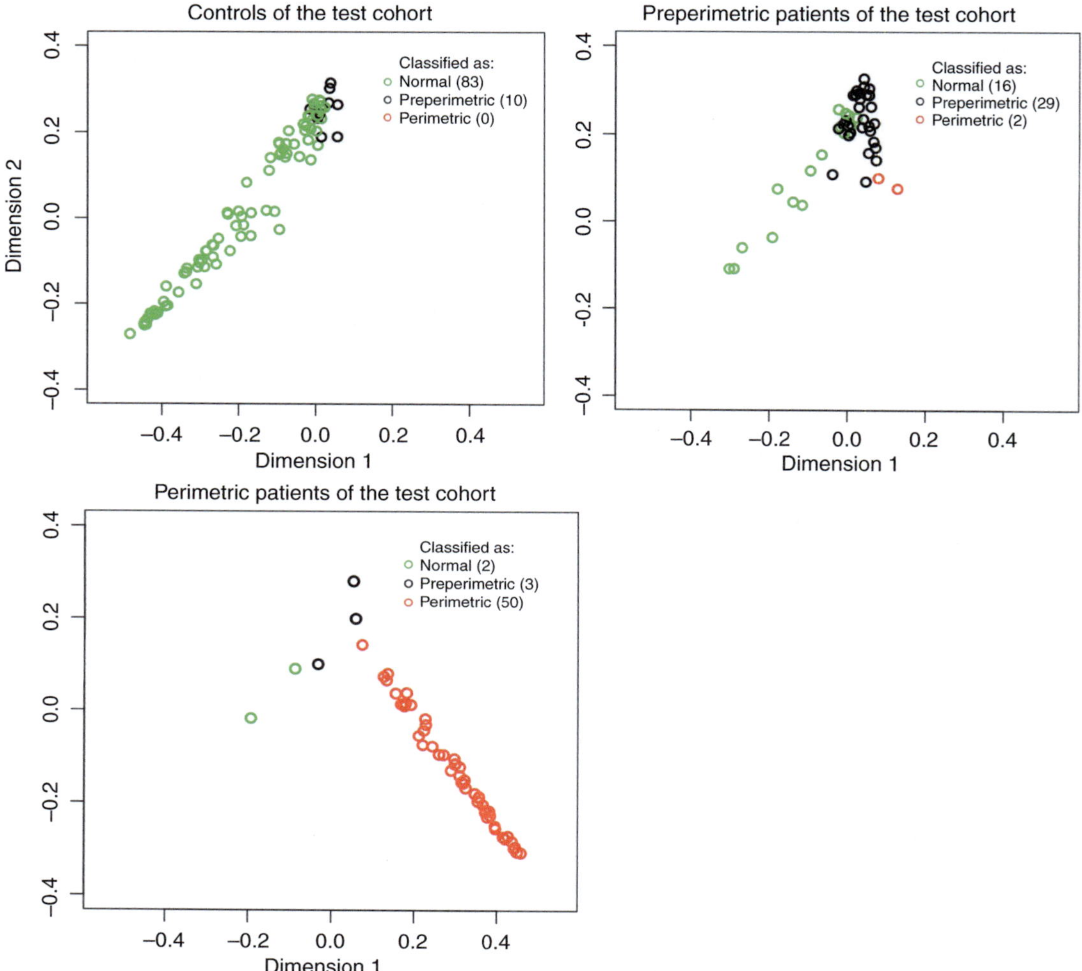

Fig. 3.5 The performance of the random forest in our test cohort is illustrated applying multidimensional scaling. The figure presents the separation between normal subjects and both patients groups. Color-coding of open symbols illustrates the class predictions of the trained random forest in groups of the test data set. Using three separate presentations of results from potential normals or pathologic eyes allows identification of outliers or misclassified subjects

position (blue ring) of this new case in the graphical multidimensional scaling plot together with the groups of our learning cohort (Fig. 3.4): controls are shown in the left part of the images in green, perimetric glaucoma patients are shown in the right part (red), and preperimetric glaucoma patients are shown in the center in black. This arrangement is very intuitive and highlights the good separation of controls from perimetric glaucomas by the random forest method. Preperimetric glaucoma patients are harder to discriminate from controls than perimetric glaucomas.

3.3.2 Results in Patients of a Test Cohort

With the trained random forest and MDS presentation, not only training data can be illustrated but also the class predictions of numerous new test data. Figure 3.5 indicates the performance of the trained classifier in subjects and patients of the university outpatient department. In contrast to Fig. 3.4, where the colors (filled symbols) indicate the real class of all subjects from the learning cohort, Fig. 3.5 illustrates the class predictions

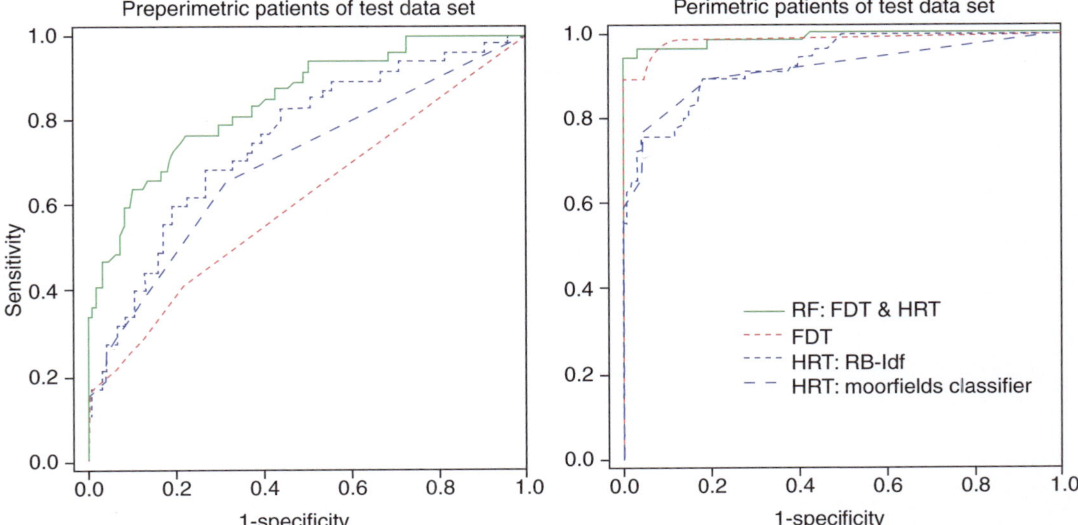

Fig. 3.6 Diagnostic value in both glaucoma groups. Receiver operating characteristic (ROC) curves illustrating the ability of the trained random forest (RF, *green lines*) to discriminate between normals and preperimetric glaucomas (*left*) and normals and perimetric glaucomas (*right*). Additionally, the performance of FDT perimetry (*dotted red lines*) and two built-in HRT classifiers (RB-ldf, Moorfields) is shown. *FDT* frequency doubling technology, *HRT* Heidelberg Retina Tomograph, *RB-ldf* built-in classifiers using linear discriminant functions. In perimetric glaucoma patients the ROC of FDT is above HRT. In early glaucomas, however, diagnostic value of HRT is larger than that of FDT. The ROC of overall analysis by random forest outperforms single test variables

by different colors for all controls and patients of the test data set. While normal subjects of our test cohort are never classified as perimetric glaucomas, ten observations are labeled preperimetric glaucomas. On the other hand, one third of the preperimetric glaucoma patients are classified as normal but only two as perimetric. The perimetric glaucoma patients could be detected quite well, with only three wrongly labeled as preperimetric glaucoma and two as normal.

The diagnostic performance of random forest in comparison to single parameter is visualized by the ROC curves for the preperimetric and perimetric patients of the present test cohort (Fig. 3.6). The areas under the ROC curves (Fig. 3.7) of the total FDT score, built-in linear discriminant functions of the HRT, and machine learning are compared. This figure includes results for a random forest trained with combined HRT and FDT parameters and with all HRT parameters only. The classification performance of the single variables of the FDT perimeter and HRT is in concordance to what we expected: the HRT performs better in the preperimetric group, and the FDT shows better results in the perimetric group. The usage of both diagnostic instruments in one machine-learning classifier combines the usefulness of each device in the preperimetric and perimetric subgroup (Fig. 3.6). The machine classifier based on all of the variables of the HRT (no FDT) is superior to all single parameter of the HRT. The discriminatory power of the multivariate parameter RB-LDF, MSD-LDF, and the corrected rim area (see Fig. 3.1) is similar in the test and learning cohort for both glaucoma groups.

3.4 Discussion

The combination of different techniques, which are able to uncover different glaucoma properties, can increase the power of a screening protocol in comparison to test with one method only. Here optic disc appearance was evaluated with scanning laser ophthalmoscopy, and sensory

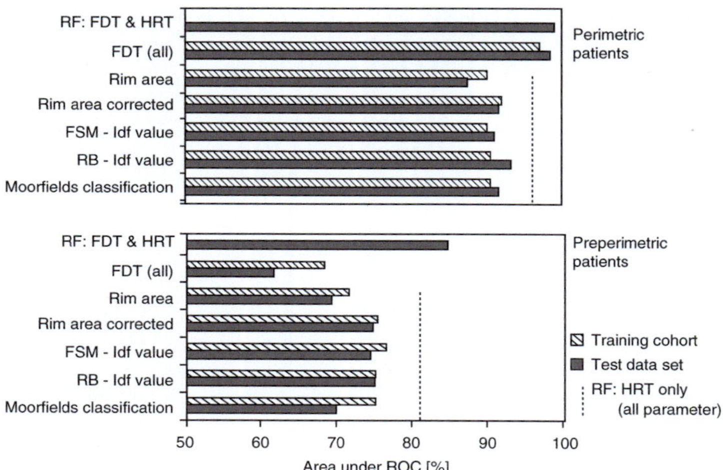

Fig. 3.7 Area under the receiver operating characteristic (ROC) curve (in %) for different diagnostic instruments in two patient groups from two independent populations: Overall score of the FDT perimeter, Moorfields classification, FSM-ldf, RB-ldf, and rim areas. In addition, the results of random forest (RF) are given when all HRT variables and the results from FDT perimetry are used in the calculation. The *vertical dotted lines* show the results of RF using the HRT variables only. *FDT* frequency doubling technology, *HRT* Heidelberg Retina Tomograph, *FSM-ldf* random forest method using the data of the learning data set, *RB-ldf* built-in classifiers using linear discriminant functions

properties were studied using the FDT perimeter. In the past HRT and FDT perimetry have been compared to each other [36–39] and with other glaucoma tests. In these comparisons, HRT and FDT perimetry competed with modern perimetric techniques [12, 40, 41] as well as with methods to inspect the nerve fiber layer [12, 42, 43]. Our FDT perimeter findings in the perimetric groups are in agreement with the results of earlier studies revealing high validity of this functional test in such patients showing losses in conventional perimetry. Considering the easy procedure and short time to perform this FDT procedure, these results recommend the method for glaucoma screening in a general population. In preperimetric glaucoma groups, however, only a small fraction of the patients has been classified glaucomatous by this functional test.

The structural method of glaucoma detection in the present evaluation uses analysis of the optic disc with scanning laser ophthalmoscopy. In the past studies have been performed to investigate the possibility of this instrument to unmask glaucomatous disc atrophy with analysis of single parameters delivered by the HRT machine as well as combinations of variables using discriminant analyses or machine-learning techniques. In these evaluations not only diagnostic value of global or sectorial measurements of the neuroretinal rim have been judged but also influence of age, sex, and the size of the optic disc have been taken into account. Measurements of optic disc variables strongly depend on the optic disc size which can vary by 1:7 [16, 36, 40, 44, 45]. In particular, assessment of large optic discs and discrimination from early glaucomatous damage is often difficult with HRT variables [46, 47]. Thus, wrong positive classification of normal optic discs increases in subjects with large optic discs, while glaucomatous small optic discs might be overlooked [35, 45, 48]. To overcome this problem and to reduce the influence of variation of neuroretinal rim and disc variability, eyes with very small or large optic discs had been excluded from earlier statistical evaluation [30, 47]. Using a multivariate equation for the correction of the neuroretinal rim area possibly allows inclusion of subjects with a larger range of optic disc size. In our patient groups, comparison between the HRT parameters indicates a diagnostic utility of the corrected rim area, which is similar, or better, to other built-in multivariate equations showing high performance (i.e., FSM-LDF, RB-LDF). It has been shown that trained neural networks, with global and regional HRT parameters used as input, can improve the discrimination between glaucomatous and nonglaucomatous eyes [49]. Similar, the present combination of 102 HRT variables with the random forest classifier is able to increase sensitivity and specificity of this device. As can be seen in Fig. 3.7, the area under the ROC curves for random forest is larger than for any of the single built-in LDF values. If the classification algorithm is learned with information from different diagnostic instruments, the technique might be able to combine their respective advantages. The diagnostic usefulness of an automated classifier has been shown recently for combination of HRT data and conventional perimetry in a study by Bowd and coworker [50]. Shah et al. [39] had investigated whether the validity of morphometric devices could be improved by additional FDT measurements and whether they could show that combined evaluation of data from FDT perimetry and HRT measurements can increase the number of correctly classified perimetric patients. Similarly, in our data, combination of output variables from both devices showed highest diagnostic performance. It should be noted that estimation of classification performance using the same data for determination of a classification rule and testing the rule leads to overoptimistic results and these estimates do not reflect the error rates that are obtained on independent test data sets or new patients. By contrast, using independently selected test data sets, unbiased estimates of the error rates are obtained. In our present study the classification formula is calculated using controls and patients with well-known class membership (controls and glaucoma patients of the Erlangen glaucoma registry) and afterward used to determine sensitivity and specificity for other subject groups. These latter subjects were members of a test population recruited independently from the reference sample.

Our results indicate that the random forest trained with HRT and FDT data is applicable as a diagnostic tool for glaucoma detection. The classifier (trained on our learning data set from the Erlangen glaucoma registry) can be requested from the authors as an R object for the inspection of personal patient data. R is available for any operating system (Windows, Linux, Mac) at no costs and can be downloaded from cran.r-project.org. Using the provided classifier, it is possible to calculate the probabilities that new observations belong to one of the three classes (normal, preperimetric, perimetric) and to create the proximity plot. The MDS plots are an easy to understand overview of the efficiency of the trained classifier. In contrast to ROC curves, they are natural illustrations of classification performance with more than two classes and allow a detection of outliers or even wrongly labeled subjects.

Conclusion

In our multimodal screening setup, we connected FDT perimetry with results from the HRT system and automatically analyzed the data with a no-cost statistical method. Using such a system, new subjects can be classified based on the data from a learning cohort with known diagnoses. The present findings not only highlight the benefit of combining functional and structural data for glaucoma detection but also show the feasibility of the application of machine-learning methods, in particular random forests. The predictive model using machine-learning classification for combination of multimodel data can be used to increase the detection rate of glaucomas.

Acknowledgments The authors thank Sylvia Rühl for skilful technical assistance; Professor G. Michelson, Professor A. Jünemann, Professor C. Mardin, and Dr. Lämmer for classification of the patients; Dipl. Ing. Dr. F. Lauterwald for implementation of the database; and Professor B. Lausen for help in statistical questions. The development of the "Erlangen Glaucoma Registry" was supported by DFG grant SFB 539. The authors have no commercial interest in the equipment used in this work.

References

1. Horn FK, Mardin CY, Bendschneider D, Junemann AG, Adler W, Tornow RP. Frequency doubling technique perimetry and spectral domain optical coherence tomography in patients with early glaucoma. Eye (Lond). 2011;25(1):17–29.
2. Johnson CA, Sample PA, Zangwill LM, Vasile CG, Cioffi GA, Liebmann JR, et al. Structure and function

evaluation (SAFE): II. Comparison of optic disk and visual field characteristics. Am J Ophthalmol. 2003; 135(2):148–54.

3. Anton A, Yamagishi N, Zangwill L, Sample PA, Weinreb RN. Mapping structural to functional damage in glaucoma with standard automated perimetry and confocal scanning laser ophthalmoscopy. Am J Ophthalmol. 1998;125(4):436–46.

4. Brigatti L, Hoffman D, Caprioli J. Neural networks to identify glaucoma with structural and functional measurements. Am J Ophthalmol. 1996;121(5):511–21.

5. Horn FK, Nguyen NX, Mardin CY, Junemann AG. Combined use of frequency doubling perimetry and polarimetric measurements of retinal nerve fiber layer in glaucoma detection. Am J Ophthalmol. 2003; 135(2):160–8.

6. Mardin CY, Peters A, Horn F, Junemann AG, Lausen B. Improving glaucoma diagnosis by the combination of perimetry and HRT measurements. J Glaucoma. 2006;15(4):299–305.

7. Racette L, Chiou CY, Hao J, Bowd C, Goldbaum MH, Zangwill LM, et al. Combining functional and structural tests improves the diagnostic accuracy of relevance vector machine classifiers. J Glaucoma. 2010; 19(3):167–75.

8. Bathija R, Zangwill L, Berry CC, Sample PA, Weinreb RN. Detection of early glaucomatous structural damage with confocal scanning laser tomography. J Glaucoma. 1998;7(2):121–7.

9. Ford BA, Artes PH, McCormick TA, Nicolela MT, LeBlanc RP, Chauhan BC. Comparison of data analysis tools for detection of glaucoma with the Heidelberg Retina Tomograph. Ophthalmology. 2003;110(6): 1145–50.

10. Mikelberg FS, Parfitt CM, Swindale NV, Graham SL, Drance SM, Gosine R. Ability of the heidelberg retina tomograph to detect early glaucomatous visual field loss. J Glaucoma. 1995;4(4):242–7.

11. Wollstein G, Garway-Heath DF, Hitchings RA. Identification of early glaucoma cases with the scanning laser ophthalmoscope. Ophthalmology. 1998; 105(8):1557–63.

12. Bowd C, Zangwill LM, Berry CC, Blumenthal EZ, Vasile C, Sanchez-Galeana C, et al. Detecting early glaucoma by assessment of retinal nerve fiber layer thickness and visual function. Invest Ophthalmol Vis Sci. 2001;42(9):1993–2003.

13. Wollstein G, Garway-Heath DF, Poinoosawmy D, Hitchings RA. Glaucomatous optic disc changes in the contralateral eye of unilateral normal pressure glaucoma patients. Ophthalmology. 2000;107(12): 2267–71.

14. Quigley HA. Identification of glaucoma-related visual field abnormality with the screening protocol of frequency doubling technology. Am J Ophthalmol. 1998; 125(6):819–29.

15. Burnstein Y, Ellish NJ, Magbalon M, Higginbotham EJ. Comparison of frequency doubling perimetry with Humphrey visual field analysis in a glaucoma practice. Am J Ophthalmol. 2000;129(3):328–33.

16. Stoutenbeek R, Heeg GP, Jansonius NM. Frequency doubling perimetry screening mode compared to the full-threshold mode. Ophthalmic Physiol Opt. 2004; 24(6):493–7.

17. Jonas JB, Gusek GC, Naumann GO. Optic disc morphometry in chronic primary open-angle glaucoma. I. Morphometric intrapapillary characteristics. Graefes Arch Clin Exp Ophthalmol. 1988;226(6): 522–30.

18. Breiman L. Bagging predictors. Mach Learn. 1996;24:123–40.

19. Lauterwald F, Neumann CP, Lenz R, Jünemann AG, Mardin CY, Meyer-Wegener K, et al. The Erlangen Glaucoma registry: a scientific database for longitudinal analysis of glaucoma. Tech Rep. 2012;CS-2011(2) :1–9. ISSN 2191-5008.

20. Jonas JB, Budde WM, Panda-Jonas S. Ophthalmoscopic evaluation of the optic nerve head. Surv Ophthalmol. 1999;43(4):293–320.

21. Horn FK, Brenning A, Junemann AG, Lausen B. Glaucoma detection with frequency doubling perimetry and short-wavelength perimetry. J Glaucoma. 2007; 16(4):363–71.

22. Casson R, James B, Rubinstein A, Ali H. Clinical comparison of frequency doubling technology perimetry and Humphrey perimetry. Br J Ophthalmol. 2001;85(3):360–2.

23. Johnson CA, Samuels SJ. Screening for glaucomatous visual field loss with frequency-doubling perimetry. Invest Ophthalmol Vis Sci. 1997;38(2):413–25.

24. Adams CW, Bullimore MA, Wall M, Fingeret M, Johnson CA. Normal aging effects for frequency doubling technology perimetry. Optom Vis Sci. 1999; 76(8):582–7.

25. Horn FK, Wakili N, Junemann AM, Korth M. Testing for glaucoma with frequency-doubling perimetry in normals, ocular hypertensives, and glaucoma patients. Graefes Arch Clin Exp Ophthalmol. 2002;240(8):658–65.

26. Hawker MJ, Vernon SA, Ainsworth G. Specificity of the Heidelberg Retina Tomograph's diagnostic algorithms in a normal elderly population: the Bridlington Eye Assessment Project. Ophthalmology. 2006;113(5):778–85.

27. Horn FK, Lammer R, Mardin CY, Junemann AG, Michelson G, Lausen B, et al. Combined evaluation of frequency doubling technology perimetry and scanning laser ophthalmoscopy for glaucoma detection using automated classification. J Glaucoma. 2012;21(1): 27–34.

28. Burk R. Laser Scanning Tomographé: Interpretation der Ausdrucke des Heidelberg Retina Tomographen HRT II [Laser scanning tomography: interpretation of the HRT II printout]. Z prakt Augenheilkd. 2001;22: 183–90.

29. Mardin CY, Horn FK. Influence of optic disc size on the sensitivity of the Heidelberg Retina Tomograph. Graefes Arch Clin Exp Ophthalmol. 1998;236(9):641–5.

30. Ramrattan RS, Wolfs RC, Jonas JB, Hofman A, de Jong PT. Determinants of optic disc characteristics in a general population: the Rotterdam Study. Ophthalmology. 1999;106(8):1588–96.

31. Mardin CY, Hothorn T, Peters A, Junemann AG, Nguyen NX, Lausen B. New glaucoma classification method based on standard Heidelberg Retina Tomograph parameters by bagging classification trees. J Glaucoma. 2003;12(4):340–6.

32. Hothorn T, Lausen B. Bagging tree classifiers for laser scanning images: a data- and simulation-based strategy. Artif Intell Med. 2003;27(1):65–79.

33. Adler W, Peters A, Lausen B. Comparison of classifiers applied to confocal scanning laser ophthalmoscopy data. Methods Inf Med. 2008;47(1):38–46.

34. Liaw A, Wiener M. Classification and regression by random forest. R News. 2002;2:18–22.

35. Borg I, Groenen P. Modern multidimensional scaling: theory and applications. New York: Springer; 1997. p. 207–12.

36. Iester M, Traverso CE, De Feo F, Sanna G, Altieri M, Vittone P, et al. Correlation between frequency doubling technology and heidelberg retina tomograph. J Glaucoma. 2005;14(5):368–74.

37. Kunimatsu S, Tomita G, Araie M, Aihara M, Suzuki Y, Iwase A, et al. Frequency doubling technology and scanning laser tomography in eyes with generalized enlargement of optic disc cupping. J Glaucoma. 2005;14(4):280–7.

38. Robin TA, Muller A, Rait J, Keeffe JE, Taylor HR, Mukesh BN. Performance of community-based glaucoma screening using Frequency Doubling Technology and Heidelberg Retinal Tomography. Ophthalmic Epidemiol. 2005;12(3):167–78.

39. Shah NN, Bowd C, Medeiros FA, Weinreb RN, Sample PA, Hoffmann EM, et al. Combining structural and functional testing for detection of glaucoma. Ophthalmology. 2006;113(9):1593–602.

40. Sample PA, Bosworth CF, Blumenthal EZ, Girkin C, Weinreb RN. Visual function-specific perimetry for indirect comparison of different ganglion cell populations in glaucoma. Invest Ophthalmol Vis Sci. 2000;41(7):1783–90.

41. Spry PG, Johnson CA, Mansberger SL, Cioffi GA. Psychophysical investigation of ganglion cell loss in early glaucoma. J Glaucoma. 2005;14(1):11–9.

42. Paczka JA, Friedman DS, Quigley HA, Barron Y, Vitale S. Diagnostic capabilities of frequency-doubling technology, scanning laser polarimetry, and nerve fiber layer photographs to distinguish glaucomatous damage. Am J Ophthalmol. 2001;131(2):188–97.

43. Landers JA, Goldberg I, Graham SL. Comparison of clinical optic disc assessment with tests of early visual field loss. Clin Experiment Ophthalmol. 2002;30(5): 338–42.

44. Agarwal HC, Gulati V, Sihota R. The normal optic nerve head on Heidelberg Retina Tomograph II. Indian J Ophthalmol. 2003;51(1):25–33.

45. Uysal Y, Bayer A, Erdurman C, Kilic S. Sensitivity and specificity of Heidelberg Retinal Tomography II parameters in detecting early and moderate glaucomatous damage: effect of disc size. Clin Experiment Ophthalmol. 2007;35(2):113–8.

46. Hoesl LM, Mardin CY, Horn FK, Juenemann AGM, Laemmer R. Influence of glaucomatous damage and optic disc size on glaucoma detection by scanning laser tomography. J Glaucoma. 2009;18(5):385–9.

47. Yip LW, Mikelberg FS. A comparison of the glaucoma probability score to earlier heidelberg retina tomograph data analysis tools in classifying normal and glaucoma patients. J Glaucoma. 2008;17(7):513–6.

48. Medeiros FA, Zangwill LM, Bowd C, Sample PA, Weinreb RN. Influence of disease severity and optic disc size on the diagnostic performance of imaging instruments in glaucoma. Invest Ophthalmol Vis Sci. 2006;47(3):1008–15.

49. Bowd C, Chan K, Zangwill LM, Goldbaum MH, Lee T-W, Sejnowski TJ, et al. Comparing neural networks and linear discriminant functions for glaucoma detection using confocal scanning laser ophthalmoscopy of the optic disc. Invest Ophthalmol Vis Sci. 2002;43(11):3444–54.

50. Bowd C, Lee I, Goldbaum MH, Balasubramanian M, Medeiros FA, Zangwill LM, et al. Predicting glaucomatous progression in glaucoma suspect eyes using relevance vector machine classifiers for combined structural and functional measurements. Invest Ophthalmol Vis Sci. 2012;53(4):2382–9.

Mass Screening of Diabetic Retinopathy Using Automated Methods

4

Michael David Abràmoff and Meindert Niemeijer

Contents

M.D. Abràmoff, MD, PhD
Retina Service, Department of Ophthalmology and Visual Sciences, Department of Electrical and Computer Engineering, Department of Biomedical Engineering, University of Iowa, 200 Hawkins Drive, PFP 11205, Iowa City, IA 52242, USA

Iowa City Veterans Medical Center, Iowa City, IA 52242, United States
e-mail: michael-abramoff@uiowa.edu

M. Niemeijer, PhD (✉)
IDx, LLC, 485 Hwy 1 West, Iowa City, IA 52246, United States
e-mail: niemeijer@eyediagnosis.net

4.1   Introduction

Regular eye examinations are necessary to diagnose diabetic retinopathy (DR) at an early stage, when it can be treated with the best prognosis and visual loss delayed or deferred [1–3]. However, compliance to these widely accepted recommendations is limited, and in 2010, in the United States, less than 60 % of the estimated 25 million people with diabetes underwent a dilated retinal examination, leaving millions of people at risk for potentially preventable visual loss and blindness [2, 4], while in the United Kingdom, with a national screening program, 74 % of people with diabetes underwent recommended screening [5].

Most screening around the world is performed by eye care providers either ophthalmologists, optometrists, or primary care physicians. Compared to the reference standard, which is dilated retinal photographs read by experienced readers, the clinical exam underperforms [6]. The sensitivity of clinicians, i.e., people with DR accurately diagnosed, as a fraction of the total number of people with DR examined, compared to such a photographic reference standard has been reported to be between 30 and 73 % in a number of studies [7–10]. The specificity, i.e., the fraction of people without DR accurately diagnosed as such during the exam, as a fraction of all without DR, was higher, between 80 and 100 % in these same studies. In addition to their limited sensitivity, another problem is the consistency of clinicians when examining patients for diabetic

G. Michelson (ed.), *Teleophthalmology in Preventive Medicine*,
DOI 10.1007/978-3-662-44975-2_4, © Springer-Verlag Berlin Heidelberg 2015

retinopathy, which is not high. For example, when reading photographs, the so-called interobserver variability of these clinicians, if not specifically trained for reading, can be poor, with κ around 0.5 [11–13].

The purpose and potential of using automated reading in screening for diabetic retinopathy is to address these issues: increasing compliance, by improving accessibility and patient friendliness through point of care assessment and decreased cost, and improving detection performance and reproducibility, by objective assessment. Typically, automated detection of DR analyzes retinal color images obtained by fundus cameras and triages those who have DR and require referral to an ophthalmologist from those who can be screened again screened again safely. The diagnostic accuracy of automated detection programs has been reported to be comparable or better than clinicians and expert readers [14–19].

This chapter will discuss the current state-of-the-art automated methods. It does not cover the various components of such methods including optic disc detection, vessel segmentation, and quality assessment, for which the reader is referred to various reviews [12, 20–22].

4.2 Goals of Automated Methods for Screening

It is crucial to be clear about the goal of automated diabetic retinopathy screening on a practical level. Because of the absence of a clinician, the goal is to identify those who need referral to an ophthalmologist for possible treatment and those who do not need such a referral. The need for referral is related to the risk of a patient with diabetic retinopathy progressing to vision loss and blindness from proliferative retinopathy, clinically significant edema, vitreous hemorrhage, or tractional detachment. These risks are different for various stages of the disease, as was established by the UK Diabetes Study, the Diabetic Retinopathy Study, and the Early Treatment for Diabetic Retinopathy Study [6, 23, 24]. These studies showed that subjects with no or mild non-proliferative retinopathy (NPDR)

and no macular edema have insufficient disease to require treatment and a low risk of advancing to treatment criteria within 1 year [6]. The risk of significant progression over several years is very low in those with no or mild NPDR without macular edema [25]. There is excellent evidence, therefore, that people with no or mild non-proliferative retinopathy levels of DR can be screened again in 1 year. The international clinical diabetic retinopathy and diabetic macular edema disease severity scales (ICDR) were proposed to capture these screening relevant stages of DR [25]. These were formulated by a consensus of international experts to standardize and simplify DR classification in order to improve communication and coordination of care among physicians caring for patients with diabetes [25]. The ICDR classification simplified the Early Treatment Diabetic Retinopathy Study (ETDRS) classification for non-proliferative and proliferative retinopathy because the latter classification had proven unwieldy in clinical care [26–29]. The ICDR defines five stages: no apparent DR, mild NPDR, moderate NPDR, severe NPDR, proliferative DR (PDR), as well as apparent macular edema present or apparent macular edema absent. Some of the proposed automated algorithms differentiate between *no and mild DR without macular edema (ME)* on the one hand and *more than mild DR or ME* on the other hand [13]. Because these designations are somewhat cumbersome, the terms referable retinopathy and diabetic eye disease (DED), respectively, have been introduced for *more than mild DR or ME*, and the term diabetic eye disease will be used in this chapter.

In the United Kingdom and Australia, which have large screening programs, a different standard, the National Screening Programme (NSP) for DR, workbook 4.3, is widely used [30]. The definitions for the various stages (R0-R3, M0, M1, P1) differ from that of the ICDR, making comparisons difficult. Approximately, R0 and R1 with M0 together are comparable to no DED, and R2 or R3 or M1 or P1 together are comparable to DED, but the details differ. However, the differences are substantial in the area where most of the disagreements between automated algorithms and human experts also occur [13]. Therefore, when sensitivity, specificity, and area under the curve are obtained from the ICDR for one automated method and from the NSP for another, these cannot be compared.

4.3 Performance and Safety of Automated Screening Methods

The first responsibility of a physician considering automated screening for DED, should be to avoid harm to the patient. A major concern of automated computer detection programs is their potential to delay diagnosis of a treatable condition. Therefore, it is important that any missed cases do not have more than moderate NPDR so that there is low risk of progression to PDR within 1 year [6]. For example, an image with a few microaneurysms only is mild NPDR, according to ICDR, but if there is one hemorrhage, it is immediately moderate NPDR, according to the ICDR. However, PDR and macular edema have a high risk of vision loss within 1 year [6], and therefore screening programs often warn people estimated to have mild DR to report promptly if they have vision loss or floaters, which possibly indicates the development of macular edema or vitreous hemorrhage from proliferative disease.

The performance of automated methods for DR screening is typically measured using sensitivity, specificity, and area under the receiver operating characteristic (ROC) curve. The sensitivity is the number of people with diabetic eye disease (DED) accurately diagnosed, as a fraction of the total number of people examined, and is a measure for the safety of the methods. A high sensitivity minimizes the number of people that are not flagged as needing additional care, while they need to. The specificity is the fraction of people without diabetic eye disease accurately diagnosed as such during the exam, as a fraction of all people without diabetic eye disease that are examined, and is a measure for the effectiveness of the method. A high specificity minimizes the number of false positives meaning that fewer people with diabetes will be referred that do not

need to be referred. Specificity is an efficiency issue that has the potential to increase productivity, and a specificity that is too low will prevent implementation [31].

There is a balance between sensitivity and specificity. It is simple to create a system with 100 % sensitivity by just diagnosing all patients examined with diabetic eye disease. Obviously such a system would not be very useful, as shown by its specificity which would be 0 %. It is just as simple to create a system with 100 % specificity, by telling all patients examined that they have no diabetic eye disease, which would not be safe, as shown by its sensitivity, which would then be 0 %. Even though most automated methods differentiate between those with and without diabetic retinopathy (of some severity), the risk of progression to vision loss is not the same for all levels of diabetic eye disease, as explained above. Someone with moderate DR according to ICDR with only the minimal criterion, a single hemorrhage, has only a 1.4 % risk of progressing to proliferative disease within 1 year, while someone with moderate DR with the maximum criteria has a 18.2 % risk of developing any proliferative disease at 1 year and a 8.5 % risk of PDR with high-risk characteristics [32]. Therefore, some studies stratify the performance by DR severity or macular edema separately, to ensure that the most severe cases have the least chance of being missed [17].

4.4 Area Under the ROC Curve and Set Point

Human experts cannot adjust their sensitivity and specificity. Automated methods usually work by calculating a number that is the likelihood of the patient having diabetic eye disease, and the final output is created by comparing this number to a so-called set point. For example, in the Iowa Detection Program, if the calculated number, called the DR Index, is larger than the set point, diabetic eye disease is called, but if it is equal or below, absence of diabetic eye disease is called [13].

A single set point leads to a single sensitivity and specificity pair. Because the set point can be changed when testing a system – but not once

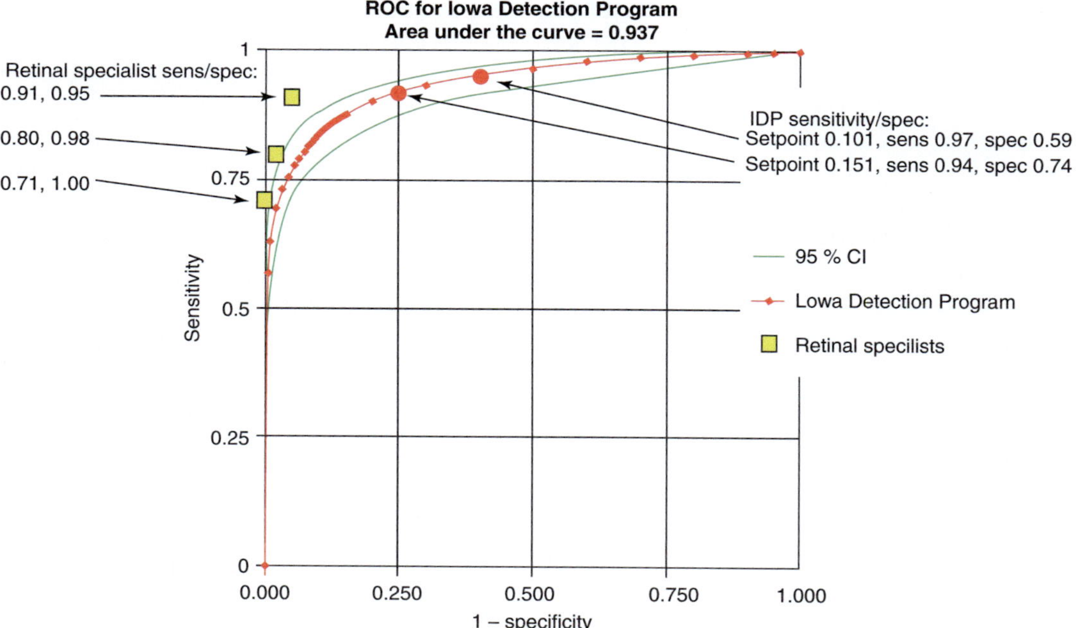

Fig. 4.1 Figure shows the receiver operating characteristic (ROC) curve for the Iowa Detection Program (IDP) as well as the sensitivity and specificity pairs of the three retinal specialists in that study for comparison. *CI* confidence interval (Adapted from Abramoff et al. [13])

is it deployed in clinical practice – different sensitivity/specificity pairs can be measured at different set points. These sensitivity/specificity pairs for a method together form its receiver operating characteristics, which can be plotted as an ROC curve. Figure 4.1 shows the ROC curve for the Iowa Detection Program as well as the sensitivity and specificity pairs of the three retinal specialists in that study for comparison.

It is hard to compare curves, and to capture the curve in a single number, the area under the ROC curve (AUC), is widely used. The AUC is a number between 0 and 1, and an automated method that is no better than a coin toss will have an AUC of 0.5, and the closer to 1 the AUC is, the better the method is able to distinguish people with diabetic eye disease from people without diabetic eye disease. A major advantage of the AUC measure is that it is not dependent on the distribution of people with and without diabetic eye disease (of some severity) in the population on which the method is tested [33]. Because the set point can be placed at a specific value, we can therefore

adjust the automated method to have an expected sensitivity and specificity. Several authors have argued that the sensitivity for detection of diabetic eye disease in a screening program is not cost effective if it is higher than 80 % or even 60 % [34]. There is some rationale for such an upper bound on sensitivity as many studies have shown that 80 % exceeds the achievable sensitivity for clinicians, which is between 30–50% [7–10]. The Australian guidelines for optometrists have in the past stated a sensitivity of 60 % [35]. If a higher sensitivity is preferred for safety reasons, for a given method, this will result in the specificity then being lower, affecting the effectiveness of the automated method as explained above. Patients or institutions, including insurance companies and governments, that pay for healthcare may opt for increased specificity at the cost of lower sensitivity, knowing that there is a low risk of missing patients who need immediate treatment, while there is a cost savings by reducing the number of people who are referred unnecessarily.

4.5 Retinal Imaging Protocols for Automated Methods

The ICDR classification does not define an imaging protocol, but does refer to the Early Treatment Diabetic Retinopathy Study (ETDRS) which was based on seven stereo photographic fields. The genesis of the ICDR was due to the fact that taking and then grading images from seven stereo fields was found to be too cumbersome to be widely used in clinical practice [25]. Previous studies have shown that reading fewer fields than seven is comparable for detecting DED to reading multiple fields or a dilated retinal examination [9, 36, 37].

Because of their relatively low cost and relative ease of use, the so-called nonmydriatic cameras, which do not require the eye to be pharmacologically dilated during focusing, are in widespread use in screening programs using human readers. The quality of the photographs is lower than the typical dilated color photos used in protocols like the ETDRS [6]. However, many studies have shown that two or even one field per eye suffices to capture most cases of diabetic eye disease, and therefore, most automated methods accept one, two, or at maximum three fields per eye at this quality level [9, 38]. Because humans can easily make a difference between a retinal image and a lens or patient label image, as required by some protocols, there is in many cases no standard order or naming convention. However, most automated methods will have unpredictable results if run on non-retinal images. Potential solutions are to use image formats or protocols that capture such meta-information, including the standard for ophthalmic fundus imaging established by the Digital Imaging Communications in Medicine (DICOM) Working Group 9 or naming conventions for the right and left eye, right and left retina, and any other structure that is imaged, so that the retinal images can be identified unequivocally without additional human input. Though formally DICOM is the standard for fundus imaging, acceptance has been slow, necessitating the latter, more involved methods.

Most cameras are fundus cameras, i.e., they measure reflectance of the retina at different wavelengths simultaneously [12]. Wide-field scanning laser ophthalmoscope (SLO) imaging is an attractive modality to image the retina, though the devices have higher cost. Recently a study of 141 people with diabetes showed that wide-field SLO read by experts had high kappas $\kappa = 0.70$ compared to the same experts reading the standard 7-field photographs [39]. However, the performance of automated methods on wide-field SLO, though in development, has not yet been published. Another potentially attractive imaging modality, optical coherence tomography (OCT) has not been validated for diabetic eye disease screening, though automated algorithms to analyze these images and potentially detect DR have been published [40].

Retinal fundus imaging with a nonmydriatic camera typically takes 10 min or more. This includes preparing the camera, discussing the procedure with the patient, accessing or recording the meta-data, and imaging both eyes. Some automated methods have their output ready in less than a minute on standard hardware [13]. This quick result can be provided at the point of care and, for most people, will eliminate the need for a separate visit to learn the result or a phone call from a healthcare professional discussing the result, thus potentially increasing compliance.

4.6 Principles of Operation of Automated Methods

Most of the automated methods discussed later in this chapter work in a similar fashion. As a typical example, the Iowa Detection Program consists of separate, mostly independent components for detecting the optic disc, fovea, and retinal vessels, measuring image quality, and detecting microaneurysms, hemorrhages, exudates, cotton wool spots, and irregular lesions including large hemorrhages and neovascularization. A fusion algorithm combines the output of all of these components into a single numerical output [13]. Examined in more detail, microaneurysm detection, one of the most important components, works by examining each pixel in each image, analyzing its color and intensity as well as that of surrounding pixels and then using these pixel level measures to group neighboring pixels into candidate lesions. Candidate lesions are then similarly analyzed on their color, size, shape, location, type, and other properties. The final output produced by the fusion algorithm is a single number, the DR Index, a dimensionless number between 0 and 1. The DR Index expresses the likelihood that the patient's images show diabetic eye disease.

Automated algorithms for microaneurysm detection were described as far back as 1984, but these analyzed angiograms, not fundus images [41]. The first microaneurysm detection algorithms were developed and evaluated by Spencer and coauthors in 1996 [42]; his method followed the standard approach of applying a sensitive candidate lesion detector followed by a classification step, and most existing microaneurysm detectors are refinements and generalizations of this approach [43, 44]. Most of the automated methods are thus considered bottom-up approaches, but an interesting exception is the University of New Mexico method developed and evaluated by Agurto and coworkers [45], who use a texture recognition approach to differentiate images with and without signs of retinopathy, a top-down approach.

4.7 Review of All Scientific Studies of Automated Methods for Mass Screening

Table 4.1 contains all studies of automated methods for diabetic eye disease screening in the scientific literature that have been evaluated on at least 300 people with diabetes [46–51]. Studies that only evaluated the performance of algorithms detecting specific lesions, as opposed to diabetic eye disease overall, were excluded, as were studies evaluating performance on only a small number of people less than 300, studies where the number of people (not images) in the tested populations could not be determined, and studies where the method required assistance by a human expert or where training data and test data were mixed. Also excluded was a study that met all of the above criteria but where some of the methods remain controversial [52, 53].

The algorithms of two groups have been evaluated multiple times, and these are indicated with a group name. Typically the differences between the different versions of these algorithms are related to the data on which they were trained and developed, the presence of additional subcomponents, and different approaches to combining the output of the different subcomponents. Because their basic approach remain similar, they are indicated with a version number, the Iowa algorithm, indicated by Iowa-0 through Iowa-3, and the Aberdeen algorithm, indicated by Aberdeen-0 to Aberdeen-2.

The measured performance of an automated method also depends on the dataset, i.e., the characteristics of the population of people with diabetes on which it is tested, the average image quality, the imaging protocol with one or more fields per eye, and the reference standard, according to which the images were read. Finally, adjudicated or voted reference standards, such as the NPS system in use in the UK screening programs are a better approximation of the truth better than a single reader. Therefore, the population and the reference standard have been indicated for each study. Because of the differences in reference standards, reading protocols and imaging protocols, it is impossible to compare the different automated methods on their absolute performance, sensitivity, and specificity. The only study comparing two different automated methods, by Abramoff and coworkers, compared an earlier version of the Iowa Detection Program (Iowa-1) and a method from the Latim group in Brest, France [15], on the same dataset read according to the same protocol. The performance on the same dataset was quite similar, and by combining the two methods, performance was improved, indicating that a combination of any of the automated methods in Table 4.1 may result in better results if compared on exactly the same test data.

Clearly, automated methods have been evaluated on large numbers of people with diabetes, the target population, and all methods achieve a sensitivity of at least 80 %, which is the minimum requirement for several countries [30]. Several of these studies have concluded that automated methods for mass screening of diabetic retinopathy are now safe [13, 17].

Table 4.1 Overview of all studies of automated methods for detecting diabetic eye disease in the scientific literature that have been evaluated on at least 300 people with diabetes. The sensitivity, specificity and area under the curve of the reported studies cannot be compared because the study methods were different.

Authors	Automated method	Year	n	Dataset	Protocol	Reference standard	Reference standard protocol	AUC	Sensitivity	Specificity	DME sensitivity	DME specificity
Abramoff [14]	Iowa-0	2008	5,692	EyeCheck (Netherlands) [46]	2×2	Single retinal specialist	EyeCheck [46]	0.84	0.84	0.64		
Abramoff [15]	Iowa-1	2010	16,670	EyeCheck (Netherlands) [46]	2×2	Single retinal specialist	EyeCheck [46]	0.84	0.90	0.48		
Abramoff [15]	Latim	2010	16,670	EyeCheck (Netherlands) [46]	2×2	Single retinal specialist	EyeCheck [46]	0.82	0.90	0.44		
Abramoff [13]	Iowa-3	2013	874	Messidor-2 (France)	2×1	3 retinal specialists adjudicated	ICDR [25]	0.94	0.97	0.59	1.00	
Agurto [45]	New Mexico	2010	822	Texas (USA)	2×3	Single retinal specialist	Texas	0.89	0.92	0.50	1.00	
Dupas [47]	Messidor-1	2010	716	Messidor-1 (France)	1×1	Single retinal specialist	Messidor		0.92	0.76	0.73	0.71
Fleming [16]	Aberdeen-1	2010	33,535	Grampian (UK)	2×1	NSP	NSP [30]		1.00	0.41	0.97	
Goatman [17]	Aberdeen-2	2011	8,271	South London (UK)	2×2	NSP	NSP [30]		0.99	0.26	0.99	
Jelinek [48]	Australia	2006	385	Australia (AUS)	2×1	Clinic (single clinician)	NSP [30]	0.93	0.85	0.90		
Philip [49]	Aberdeen-0	2007	6,722	Grampian (UK)	2×1	NSP	NSP [30]		0.91	0.67		
Sanchez [50]	Iowa-2	2011	1,200	Messidor-1 (France)	1×1	Single reader	EyeCheck [48]	0.88	0.92	0.50		
Usher [51]	St. George	2004	773	London (UK)	1×1	Single reader	NICE/EURODIAB		0.95	0.46		

n number of people included in the study dataset, *Protocol* imaging protocol indicated by number of eyes × number of fields, all studies used non-stereo images, *AUC* area under receiver operator characteristics curve, sensitivity, and specificity for diabetic eye disease overall, DME sensitivity indicates sensitivity to detect diabetic macular edema, if this separate performance is provided, *DME* diabetic macular edema, *ICDR* international clinical diabetic retinopathy and diabetic macular edema disease severity scales, *NSP* National Screening Programme

Conclusion

Automated methods for mass screening of diabetic eye disease have matured to a safety level that merits considering deployment in clinical practice provided all regulatory criteria are met. Before introducing an automated method, goals of the screening program, imaging protocols, and risks should be carefully understood and their relative merits considered. In other words, there is accumulating evidence that automated methods for detecting diabetic eye disease are poised to increase the number of people with diabetes screened, decrease the cost per person screened, and reduce vision loss caused by delayed treatment.

References

1. Bragge P, Gruen RL, Chau M, Forbes A, Taylor HR. Screening for presence or absence of diabetic retinopathy: a meta-analysis. Arch Ophthalmol. 2011;129(4):435–44.
2. Hazin R, Colyer M, Lum F, Barazi MK. Revisiting diabetes 2000: challenges in establishing nationwide diabetic retinopathy prevention programs. Am J Ophthalmol. 2011;152(5):723–9.
3. National Health Services, The English Diabetic Eye Screening Programme (United Kingdom). The NHS diabetic retinopathy programme: Annual report, 1 April 2007–31 March 2008. Gloucester: Gloucestershire Hospitals NHS Trust and the English National Health Service; 2008 [cited 2014 Oct 10]. http://diabeticeye. screening.nhs.uk/getdata.php?id=10858.
4. Centers for Disease Control and Prevention. National diabetes fact sheet: national estimates and general information on diabetes and prediabetes in the United States. Atlanta: U.S. Department of Health and Human Services, Centers for Disease Control and Prevention; 2008.
5. National Health Services Diabetic Eye Screening Programme (United Kingdom);. Facts and Figures. Gloucester: NHS Diabetic Eye Screening Programme. 2013 [cited 2014 Oct 10]. http://diabeticeye.screening.nhs.uk/statistics.
6. Fundus photographic risk factors for progression of diabetic retinopathy. ETDRS report number 12. Early Treatment Diabetic Retinopathy Study Research Group. Ophthalmology. 1991;98(5 Suppl):823–33.
7. Pugh JA, Jacobson JM, Van Heuven WA, Watters JA, Tuley MR, Lairson DR. Screening for diabetic retinopathy. The wide-angle retinal camera. Diabetes Care. 1993;16(6):889–95.
8. Lawrence MG. The accuracy of digital-video retinal imaging to screen for diabetic retinopathy: an analysis of two digital-video retinal imaging systems using standard stereoscopic seven-field photography and dilated clinical examination as reference standards. Trans Am Ophthalmol Soc. 2004;102:321–40.
9. Lin DY, et al. The sensitivity and specificity of single-field nonmydriatic monochromatic digital fundus photography with remote image interpretation for diabetic retinopathy screening: a comparison with ophthalmoscopy and standardized mydriatic color photography. Am J Ophthalmol. 2002;134(2):204–13.
10. Emanuele N, Klein R, Moritz T, Davis MD, Glander K, Anderson R, et al. Comparison of dilated fundus examinations with seven-field stereo fundus photographs in the Veterans Affairs Diabetes Trial. J Diabetes Complications. 2009;23(5):323–9.
11. Ruamviboonsuk P, Teerasuwanajak K, Tiensuwan M, Yuttitham K, Thai Screening for Diabetic Retinopathy Study Group. Interobserver agreement in the interpretation of single-field digital fundus images for diabetic retinopathy screening. Ophthalmology. 2006;113(5):826–32.
12. Abramoff MD, Garvin M, Sonka M. Retinal imaging and image analysis. IEEE Rev Biomed Eng. 2010;3:169–208.
13. Abràmoff MD, Folk JC, Han DP, Walker JD, Williams DF, Russell SR, et al. Automated analysis of retinal images for detection of referable diabetic retinopathy. JAMA Ophthalmol. 2013;131(3):351–7.
14. Abràmoff MD, Niemeijer M, Suttorp-Schulten MS, Viergever MA, Russell SR, van Ginneken B. Evaluation of a system for automatic detection of diabetic retinopathy from color fundus photographs in a large population of patients with diabetes. Diabetes Care. 2008;31(2):193–8.
15. Abràmoff MD, Reinhardt JM, Russell SR, Folk JC, Mahajan VB, Niemeijer M, et al. Automated early detection of diabetic retinopathy. Ophthalmology. 2010;117(6):1147–54.
16. Fleming AD, Goatman KA, Philip S, Prescott GJ, Sharp PF, Olson JA. Automated grading for diabetic retinopathy: a large-scale audit using arbitration by clinical experts. Br J Ophthalmol. 2010;94(12):1606–10.
17. Goatman K, Charnley A, Webster L, Nussey S. Assessment of automated disease detection in diabetic retinopathy screening using two-field photography. PLoS One. 2011;6(12):27524.
18. Scotland GS, McNamee P, Fleming AD, Goatman KA, Philip S, Prescott GJ, et al. Costs and consequences of automated algorithms versus manual grading for the detection of referable diabetic retinopathy. Br J Ophthalmol. 2010;94(6):712–9.
19. Scotland GS, McNamee P, Philip S, Fleming AD, Goatman KA, Prescott GJ, et al. Cost-effectiveness of implementing automated grading within the national screening programme for diabetic retinopathy in Scotland. Br J Ophthalmol. 2007;91(11):1518–23.
20. Niemeijer M, van Ginneken B, Cree MJ, Mizutani A, Quellec G, Sanchez CI, et al. Retinopathy online challenge: automatic detection of microaneurysms in digital color fundus photographs. IEEE Trans Med Imaging. 2010;29(1):185–95.
21. Winder RJ, Morrow PJ, McRitchie IN, Bailie JR, Hart PM. Algorithms for digital image processing in

diabetic retinopathy. Comput Med Imaging Graph. 2009;33(8):608–22.

22. Teng T, Lefley M, Claremont D. Progress towards automated diabetic ocular screening: a review of image analysis and intelligent systems for diabetic retinopathy. Med Biol Eng Comput. 2002;40(1): 2–13.

23. Four risk factors for severe visual loss in diabetic retinopathy. The third report from the Diabetic Retinopathy Study. The Diabetic Retinopathy Study Research Group. Arch Ophthalmol. 1979;97(4): 654–5.

24. Kohner EM, Aldington SJ, Stratton IM, Manley SE, Holman RR, Matthews DR, et al. United Kingdom Prospective Diabetes Study, 30: diabetic retinopathy at diagnosis of non-insulin-dependent diabetes mellitus and associated risk factors. Arch Ophthalmol. 1998;116(3):297–303.

25. Wilkinson CP, Ferris 3rd FL, Klein RE, Lee PP, Agardh CD, Davis M, et al. Proposed international clinical diabetic retinopathy and diabetic macular edema disease severity scales. Ophthalmology. 2003; 110(9):1677–82.

26. Photocoagulation for diabetic macular edema. Early Treatment Diabetic Retinopathy Study report number 1. Early Treatment Diabetic Retinopathy Study research group. Arch Ophthalmol. 1985;103(12):1796–806.

27. Nguyen QD, Brown DM, Marcus DM, Boyer DS, Patel S, Feiner L, et al. Ranibizumab for diabetic macular edema: results from 2 phase III randomized trials: RISE and RIDE. Ophthalmology. 2012;119(4): 789–801.

28. Mitchell P, Bandello F, Schmidt-Erfurth U, Lang GE, Massin P, Schlingemann RO, et al. The RESTORE study: ranibizumab monotherapy or combined with laser versus laser monotherapy for diabetic macular edema. Ophthalmology. 2011;118(4):615–25.

29. Diabetic Retinopathy Clinical Research Network, et al. Randomized trial evaluating ranibizumab plus prompt or deferred laser or triamcinolone plus prompt laser for diabetic macular edema. Ophthalmology. 2010;117(6):1064–77.e35.

30. National Screening Programme for Diabetic Retinopathy Workbook 4.3, updated 2009. UK National Screening Committee.

31. Kocher R, Sahni N. Rethinking health care labor. N Engl J Med. 2011;365:1370–2.

32. Davis MD, Fisher MR, Gangnon RE, Barton F, Aiello LM, Chew EY, et al. Risk factors for high-risk proliferative diabetic retinopathy and severe visual loss: Early Treatment Diabetic Retinopathy Study Report #18. Invest Ophthalmol Vis Sci. 1998;39(2): 233–52.

33. McNeil BJ, Hanley JA. Statistical approaches to the analysis of receiver operating characteristic (ROC) curves. Med Decis Making. 1984;4(2):137–50.

34. Javitt JC, Canner JK, Sommer A. Cost effectiveness of current approaches to the control of retinopathy in type I diabetics. Ophthalmology. 1989;96(2): 255–64.

35. National Health and Medical Research Council (Australia). Clinical Practice Guidelines: Management of Diabetic Retinopathy. Canberra, Australia: NHMRC; 1997 [cited 2010 Oct.10]. http://www.nhmrc.gov.au/_ files_nhmrc/publications/attachments/cp53.pdf.

36. Ahmed J, Ward TP, Bursell SE, Aiello LM, Cavallerano JD, Vigersky RA. The sensitivity and specificity of nonmydriatic digital stereoscopic retinal imaging in detecting diabetic retinopathy. Diabetes Care. 2006;29(10):2205–9.

37. Cavallerano JD, Aiello LP, Cavallerano AA, Katalinic P, Hock K, Kirby R, et al. Nonmydriatic digital imaging alternative for annual retinal examination in persons with previously documented no or mild diabetic retinopathy. Am J Ophthalmol. 2005;140(4): 667–73.

38. Chew EY. Screening options for diabetic retinopathy. Curr Opin Ophthalmol. 2006;17(6):519–22.

39. Kernt M, et al. Assessment of diabetic retinopathy using nonmydriatic ultra-widefield scanning laser ophthalmoscopy (Optomap) compared with ETDRS 7-field stereo photography. Diabetes Care. 2012;35(12):2459–63.

40. Sohn EH, Chen JJ, Lee K, Niemeijer M, Sonka M, Abràmoff MD. Reproducibility of diabetic macular edema estimates from SD-OCT is affected by the choice of image analysis algorithm. Invest Ophthalmol Vis Sci. 2013;54(6):4184–8.

41. Baudoin CE, Lay BJ, Klein JC. Automatic detection of microaneurysms in diabetic fluorescein angiography. Rev Epidemiol Sante Publique. 1984;32(3–4):254–61.

42. Spencer T, Olson JA, McHardy KC, Sharp PF, Forrester JV. An image-processing strategy for the segmentation and quantification of microaneurysms in fluorescein angiograms of the ocular fundus. Comput Biomed Res. 1996;29(4):284–302.

43. Niemeijer M, van Ginneken B, Staal J, Suttorp-Schulten MS, Abràmoff MD. Automatic detection of red lesions in digital color fundus photographs. IEEE Trans Med Imaging. 2005;24(5):584–92.

44. Fleming AD, Philip S, Goatman KA, Olson JA, Sharp PF. Automated microaneurysm detection using local contrast normalization and local vessel detection. IEEE Trans Med Imaging. 2006;25(9):1223–32.

45. Agurto C, Barriga ES, Murray V, Nemeth S, Crammer R, Bauman W, et al. Automatic detection of diabetic retinopathy and age-related macular degeneration in digital fundus images. Invest Ophthalmol Vis Sci. 2011;52(8):5862–71.

46. Abramoff MD, Suttorp-Schulten MS. Web-based screening for diabetic retinopathy in a primary care population: the EyeCheck project. Telemed J E Health. 2005;11(6):668–74.

47. Dupas B, et al. Evaluation of automated fundus photograph analysis algorithms for detecting microaneurysms, haemorrhages and exudates, and of a computer-assisted diagnostic system for grading diabetic retinopathy. Diabetes Metab. 2010;36(3): 213–20.

48. Jelinek HJ, et al. An automated microaneurysm detector as a tool for identification of diabetic retinopathy

in rural optometric practice. Clin Exp Optom. 2006; 89(5):299–305.

49. Philip S, Fleming AD, Goatman KA, Fonseca S, McNamee P, Scotland GS, et al. The efficacy of automated "disease/no disease" grading for diabetic retinopathy in a systematic screening programme. Br J Ophthalmol. 2007;91(11):1512–7.

50. Sánchez CI, Niemeijer M, Dumitrescu AV, Suttorp-Schulten MS, Abràmoff MD, van Ginneken B. Evaluation of a computer-aided diagnosis system for diabetic retinopathy screening on public data. Invest Ophthalmol Vis Sci. 2011;52:4866–71.

51. Usher D, Dumskyj M, Himaga M, Williamson TH, Nussey S, Boyce J. Automated detection of diabetic retinopathy in digital retinal images: a tool for diabetic retinopathy screening. Diabet Med. 2004;21(1): 84–90.

52. Fleming AD, Olson JA, Sharp PF, Goatman KA, Philip S. Response to 'Improved automated screening of diabetic retinopathy' by Carlos M Oliveira et al. Ophthalmologica. 2012;227(3):173; author reply 174.

53. Oliveira CM, Cristóvão LM, Ribeiro ML, Abreu JR. Improved automated screening of diabetic retinopathy. Ophthalmologica. 2011;226(4):191–7.

Low-Cost Non-mydriatic Color Video Imaging of the Retina for Nonindustrialized Countries

5

Bernhard Höher, Georg Michelson,
Peter Voigtmann, and Bernhard Schmauss

Contents

B. Höher, Dipl.-Ing (✉)
Department of Electrical Engineering,
Lehrstuhl für Hochfrequenztechnik,
Cauerstr. 9, 91058 Erlangen, Germany

Institute of Microwaves and Photonics, University
of Erlangen Nuremberg, Erlangen, Germany
e-mail: bernhard.hoeher@fau.de

G. Michelson, MD
Department of Ophthalmology, Interdisciplinary
Center of Ophthalmic Preventive Medicine
and Imaging, Friedrich-Alexander University
Erlangen-Nürnberg, Erlangen, Germany
e-mail: Georg.michelson@uk-erlangen.de

P. Voigtmann, Dipl.-Kfm
Voigtmann GmbH, Nürnberg, Germany
e-mail: pv@voigtmann.de

B. Schmauss, Dr.-Ing
Institute of Microwaves and Photonics, University
of Erlangen Nuremberg, Erlangen, Germany
e-mail: Bernhard.Schmauss@fau.de

5.1   Introduction

Viewing and photographing the fundus of the human eye is an important diagnosis method in ophthalmology. It offers the chance for an early diagnosis of diabetic retinopathy, age-related macular degeneration, and many other diseases of the eye. The cost of fundus cameras is typically about 20,000–50,000 US$. As a consequence many fundus cameras are not available for developing countries. However, especially for those countries there is a need for fundus cameras within telemedical applications, because medical doctors often are not available in rural areas.

Our aim was to design a fundus camera offering an optimal compromise between costs, image quality, robustness, and ease of use and to improve the technology itself by investigation.

To find a proper imaging technology, we first decided between the two major types of fundus cameras: scanning laser ophthalmoscopes (SLOs)

G. Michelson (ed.), *Teleophthalmology in Preventive Medicine*,
DOI 10.1007/978-3-662-44975-2_5, © Springer-Verlag Berlin Heidelberg 2015

and classic color fundus cameras. As SLOs are expensive and technically more complex with many damageable mechanically moving parts, we decided to use the classical non-scanning approach. Thus, only non-scanning devices are considered in the further discussion.

Many color fundus cameras depend on an artificially dilated pupil making this method invasive. Non-mydriatic fundus cameras on the market can acquire images at smaller pupils without the use of mydriatic substances. Many of them have a severe disadvantage: They still need a pupil size of at least 4 mm typically. As a consequence the pupil has to be naturally dilated by darkened examination rooms. Furthermore, the pupil will shrink after taking a fundus image as a reaction on the flashlight of the fundus camera. Thus, there is a certain time span of typically a few minutes that has to be waited until the pupil has widened up again to take another fundus image. Therefore, typical non-mydriatic fundus cameras are not able to take images in quick succession or videos. We investigated on the imaging technology to acquire fundus images even at pupil sizes down to 2 mm to take fundus images at non-dilated eyes and to acquire videos.

5.2   Imaging Method

Imaging with a wide angle of view is challenging in optics, because many optical imaging errors get worse with an increasing angle to the optical axis. Far-reaching skills and experience in optical lens design are necessary to design such wide-field lenses with low aberrations. To avoid reengineering of existing technology, the design of the fundus camera was performed as a combination of standard problems. For those standard problems in optical engineering, there are several ready-to-use solutions available on the market. Those solutions are reliable, established, optimized, and inexpensive. This reduced the effort in engineering and enabled the use of low-cost but well-optimized mass-market components. There were two standard solutions being combined: first to generate an intermediate image of the retina and second to project this intermediate image to a CCD (charge-coupled device).

The first step was solved by an eyepiece intended for amateur astronomy. Such eyepieces originally are intended to project the intermediate image of a telescope onto the retina. The field of view is a main feature that is advertised in the market of astronomical eyepieces. Therefore, relatively cheap eyepieces with a large field of view up to 100° and above are available. However, the imaging quality at the periphery is lower than in the center. Therefore, an eyepiece with 68° field of view was used with costs of only about 150 US$. By using this eyepiece in the opposite direction for funduscopy, a 68° angle of view onto the retina could be gained.

The second step was to project the intermediate image onto a CCD. Therefore, a photographic C-mount lens intended for industry applications was used. The cost of such a photographic lens is about 250 US$.

Both components (eyepiece and photographic lens) were optically matched by a field lens. This was necessary to adapt the different apertures. Therefore, an achromatic lens (110 US$) was used.

To increase the image quality and to reduce light stress to the subject, a monochrome CCD was used, as monochrome CCDs are more light sensitive compared to color CCDs. Thus, the light energy being necessary for a given image quality is reduced. Nevertheless, color images are generated even with a monochrome CCD by using a special illumination method.

5.3   Illumination Method

A special illumination technique was applied to generate color images in spite of using a monochrome CCD [1, 2]. This was achieved by acquiring three monochrome images sequentially, each image illuminated with one of the three primary colors: red, green, and blue. Subsequently the three monochrome images were digitally superimposed by additive color mixing to get one color image. The advantage of this method was that there is no loss of light at the color filters that would have been in front of the pixels of a color CCD. Therefore, the light energy being necessary for a given image quality was reduced.

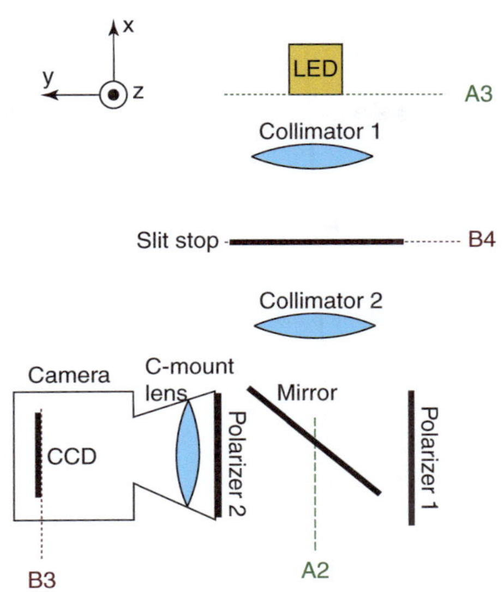

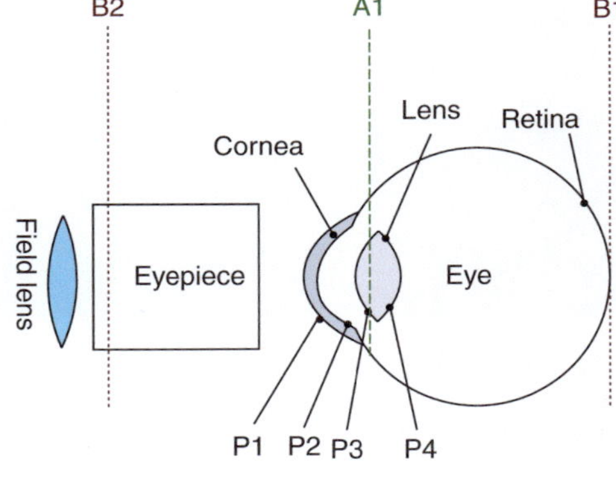

Fig. 5.1 Top view of the optical design (z-axis is vertical)

Furthermore, this sequential method offered the flexibility to create false-color or multispectral images including infrared and ultraviolet wavelengths. The images can be registered (aligned) to coincide with each other at the color mixing step. However, the registering step was not needed between saccades, when the eye was still.

This color illumination was realized by using a power LED (light-emitting diode) module, which contained three emitters with the colors red, green, and blue. The emitters were sequentially switched on by a microcontroller being synchronized by the strobe control line of the CCD camera. The length and the order of the color sequence were arbitrarily adjustable. For example, it could be switched to a red-free mode easily without adding any expensive optical filters. Instead the red emitter was just switched off.

A system of two collimators projected the LED to a mirror resulting in a downsized image of the LED. This downsized image of the LED worked as a virtual light source. This light source at the aperture plane A2 (Fig. 5.1) is projected to the aperture plane A1 located in the pupil of the eye. This second projection by the eyepiece performs another downscaling of the LED image. By

this method a very small virtual light source was generated in the pupil of the eye, so that the illumination light bundle passed the pupil with a very narrow waist. Behind the pupil the light bundle diverged and illuminated a stripe-shaped area of the retina. This square area (18° by 68°) defined the field of view. The special shape of the field was needed for reflection suppression methods.

5.4 Suppression of Back Reflections

A challenging part at the design of a non-mydriatic fundus camera is the reduction of back reflections at optical surfaces. Those reflections can occur wherever the illuminating and observing light bundles interfere [3]. In our design this affects the field lens, the eyepiece, the cornea, and the lens of the eye. Back reflections within the eye occur at four surfaces, which are tagged with P1 to P4 in Fig. 5.1. They are causing the so-called Purkinje image nos. 1 to 4, respectively [4].

Without any further measures, it would not have been possible to acquire fundus images by the described way, because the back reflections

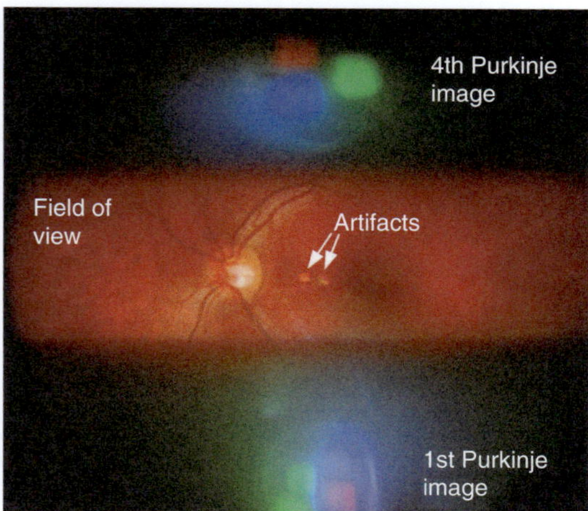

Fig. 5.2 Stripe-field method: reflections focused to unused *upper/lower black stripes*, gaining unlimited width of the field of view in the center

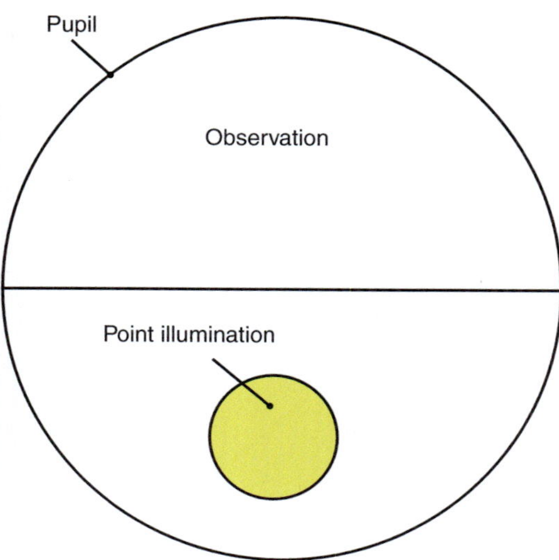

Fig. 5.3 Bisection of the aperture: separation of illumination from observation for suppression of the 1st and 2nd Purkinje reflections

would be many magnitudes brighter than the fundus image. Thus, several measures to reduce those back reflections were applied.

The first measure was to use an eyepiece and a field lens with an antireflection coating. For eyepieces this is a standard feature, which is included for nearly all products on the market. However, there are still remaining reflections, which are still too bright. Of course the eye does not have such a coating on its optical surfaces, too.

Therefore, another measure using polarized light [5] was applied. This means that one polarizer is put in front of the virtual light source in plane A2 (Fig. 5.1) and another one in front of the C-mount lens. The polarizing filters were relatively axially turned by 90° ("crossed"). As a consequence no light from the illumination could enter the camera as long as the polarization of the light was not changed. The field lens and the eyepiece did not change the state of polarization of the light, so that back reflections at their surfaces were nearly completely suppressed. Only small artifacts remained (Fig. 5.2), which could be suppressed by image post-processing, because they were reproducible. The Purkinje images were reduced in intensity, too, but the effectiveness decreased with the increasing number of the Purkinje reflection. This was due to birefringence within the cornea and lens, which changed the state of polarization.

Finally the light was scattered on the retina, which depolarized the illuminating light so that an orthogonal polarization component was generated passing the second polarizer.

To suppress the Purkinje images, the light bundles of illumination and observation were separated at the aperture plane A1 (Fig. 5.1) [3, 6]. The position of this aperture plain was settled near the front side of the lens of the eye. Figure 5.3 shows the bisection of the aperture plane A1 to an upper observation section and a lower illumination spot. This prevented the disturbing rays, being reflected at the cornea or lens, from mixing up with the useful rays emerging from the retina.

The suppression of Purkinje images by aperture splitting only can work perfectly at the aperture plane itself. However, the origins of the Purkinje images are located at the cornea or lens and therefore have some axial distance to the aperture plane. Depending on this distance, the illuminating and observing ray bundles interfered more or less. Thus, the Purkinje images (especially the 1st and 4th) could be suppressed partially only.

To overcome this problem, a new method was found: The optics were designed in a way that the 1st and 4th Purkinje images were not blurred over the whole fundus image, but focused to peripheral areas of the image plane. The remaining space between the 1st and 4th Purkinje images was free of artifacts and was used for imaging. Therefore, a stripe-shaped field of view was used, because it fitted in between the reflections (Fig. 5.2). There is an important difference between the described stripe-field method and stripe aperture devices as described in the literature [7] or other devices based on slit lamps. In those devices the aperture plane and not the image plane is divided into stripes.

Thus, the stripe-field method combined with the other measures being described makes it possible to capture wide-field fundus images being free of reflections and artifacts.

5.5   Video Capability with a Large Field of View

Many conventional non-mydriatic fundus cameras use a ring illumination, which is different from our stripe-field method. The main disadvantage of conventional ring illumination is that the field of view decreases with a decreasing pupil diameter. For example, when the pupil shrinks down to 1.58 mm, the possible field of view is only 20° [8]. This is why many common fundus cameras with 45° field of view normally need at least about 4 mm pupil diameter to work properly. Some cameras offer a small pupil mode with a reduced field of view. This shows the correlation between pupil diameter and maximum field of view. This is a major problem of that method, because after activating the illumination, the pupil will quickly shrink below the critical diameter. Therefore, the ring illumination cannot be continuous, but must be "flashed" to quickly capture an image before the pupil shrinks. If another image has to be taken, one has to wait up to some minutes until the pupil has enlarged above the limit again. At permanent illumination, which is required for video acquisition, the pupil would shrink down to about 1.5–2 mm, resulting in a field of view of only about 20°.

Our stripe-field illumination method solved the described small pupil problem. The advance in the method was that the rotational symmetry of the ring illumination was left. The square field of view

offered the two parameters height and width of the field of view. Those parameters were two degrees of freedom being available for optimization. This is one parameter more compared to the conventional ring illumination where only the diameter could be optimized. This was used to load all the "small pupil problems," which reduced the maximum angle of view, to the vertical axis, leaving the horizontal axis free of those problems. This means that the height of our image was still limited by the pupil size to about 20° like it is at ring illumination, but the width of the fundus image became unlimited in principle. Practically the width of the field could be extended as far as the eyepiece can afford. Thus, the new method allowed a continuous illumination of the fundus while still having a wide-field and artifactless view to the fundus. This offered the possibility to acquire wide-field videos. Furthermore, if only one still image were needed, then many video frames could be averaged by post-processing to drastically increase the clarity (see below).

5.6   Positioning of the Fundus Camera

Especially for non-mydriatic fundus cameras, it is necessary to correctly align the camera to the eye, because the very small pupil has to be targeted and does not left much space for misalignments. Therefore, an accurate positioning method was essential for a reliable operation. Fortunately, our stripe-field imaging method offered the complimentary feature for pupil tracking in three dimensions without the need for any further design features in hardware. This was achieved by taking advantage of the Purkinje images (especially image nos. 1 and 4) above and below the field of view, which are also captured by the CCD (Fig. 5.2). The position and shape of those reflections sensitively revealed a displacement of the device in all three spatial dimensions. Figure 5.4a shows the Purkinje images at a correct alignment and also at a displacement in each of the three spatial directions (Fig. 5.4b–d). The operator of the fundus camera was able to align the camera to the subject continuously by watching the reflections on the live preview of the control software.

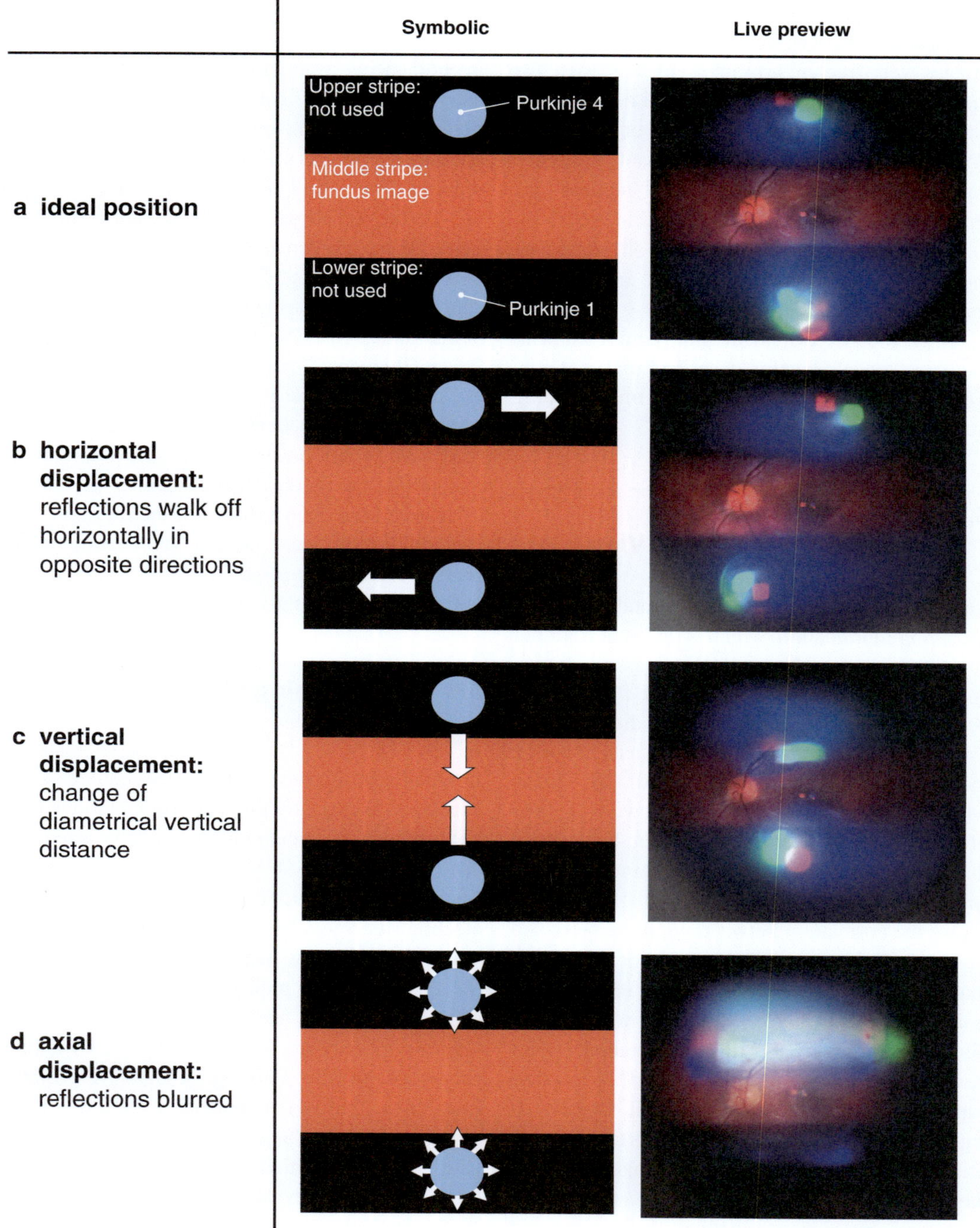

Fig. 5.4 Positioning method by Purkinje reflections: signs of displacement seen by the operator at the live preview. (**a**) *Ideal positions*; (**b**) *horizontal displacement*, reflections walk off horizontally in opposite directions; (**c**) *vertical displacement*, change of diametrical vertical distance; and (**d**) *axial displacement*, reflections blurred

At a horizontal misalignment, the reflections were not arranged in a vertical line (Fig. 5.4b). The vertical position of the device changed the distance between the Purkinje images. If the device was located too high, the reflections walked into the image (Fig. 5.4c). If it was too low, the illumination left the pupil resulting in a loss of illumination. Therefore, the operator moved the fundus camera vertically until the Purkinje reflections were located just outside of the middle stripe. If the device was misaligned axially, then the reflections were blurred (Fig. 5.4d). By this effect the operator was able to adjust the ideal distance of the camera to the subject precisely until the reflections became clear. The areas outside the field of view were only useful for positioning. Thus, the images were cropped for further processing steps.

The manual tracking by the operator worked well. It is promising that an automatic position guider based on the Purkinje reflections would also work well; however, it was not worked on this, yet. Future works may prove this.

5.7 Waiver of Handheld Operation

Several handheld fundus cameras are described in the literature [9–11]. Handheld operation would also be possible with our fundus camera, because of its small dimensions. However, it was explicitly decided against handheld operation, because the experience was made that non-mydriatic fundus cameras are not practicable for handheld operation, because of the very small dimension of the pupil, which needs a high positioning accuracy. Normally an operator was not able to target an undilated pupil with the needed submillimeter accuracy. It revealed that good images were just a matter of chance in handheld operation. Only with trained subjects, it was possible to get at least a small percentage of usable images. However, when the subject was kept still by the commonly used chin and forehead rests, a reliable operation could be gained. Furthermore, the fundus camera was mounted on a modified positioning unit of a slit lamp to align the camera with a high precision.

It is obvious that an accurate positioning is essential for any non-mydriatic fundus camera with any imaging method, because the fundus camera just cannot "look" into the eye if it is not properly targeted to the very small pupil. Thus, the fixation unit for the subject and the fine positioning unit revealed as essential components of our non-mydriatic fundus camera. Without them a reliable operation could not be guaranteed.

It is questionable if it is possible to design a handheld device that enables a good fixation of the subject and a fine positioning. From our experience we believe that good fixation and fine positioning are not possible with a handheld device for the most operators and subjects.

5.8 Realization and Evaluation of a Demonstrator

A mobile demonstrator [12] was realized to evaluate the described stripe-field method (Figs. 5.5 and 5.6). An eyepiece with a focal length of 21 mm and a CCD camera (sensor: Sony ICX274, $1{,}628 \times 1{,}236$ pixel) including a C-mount lens ($f = 16$ mm) with a motorized focus was used. Spherical refractive errors from $+10$ to -10 dpt could be compensated by a focus slider within the control software of the fundus camera. This is realized by a motor in the fundus camera moving the photographic lens. This is the only moving part within the fundus camera; otherwise, it is a solid-state device making it very robust. The illumination was realized by a triple LED with dominant emission wavelengths of 625 nm (red), 527 nm (green), and 470 nm (blue) each having an electrical power of 1 W. It was important to get the unmodified raw data of the images to enable a scientific evaluation of the methods. Therefore, a gigabit Ethernet interface was used to transmit the immense data volume to a PC. The data was recorded by a special PC application, programmed with C++, which was also used to

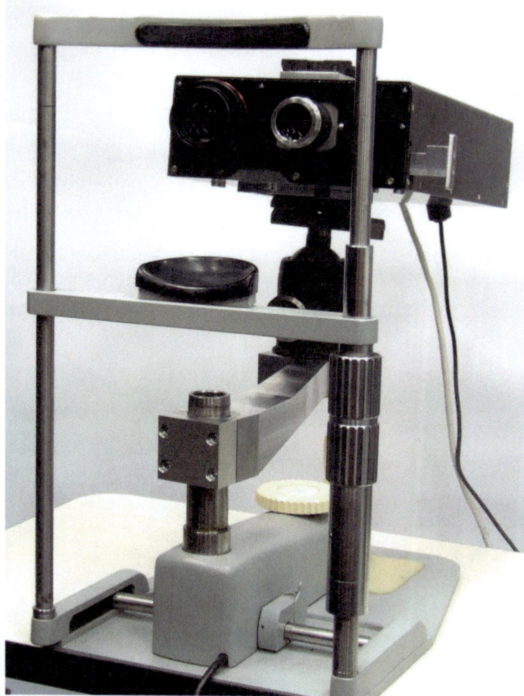

Fig. 5.5 Lab demonstrator: non-mydriatic fundus video camera with 68° × 18° field of view mounted on a modified positioning unit of a slit lamp

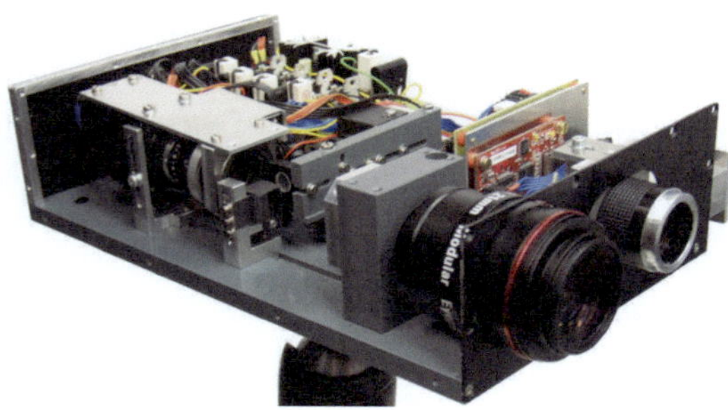

Fig. 5.6 Lab demonstrator without casing box

control the fundus camera via a microcontroller and to display a live preview. The weight of the device (without the chin rest) was only 2.8 kg and the outer dimensions were 30 × 20 × 8 cm. The cost of the lab demonstrator as single-piece production was around 5,000 US$.

5.9 Image Post-processing

The image quality was enhanced by several digital image processing steps. Figure 5.7 shows the fundus of a 23-year-old healthy male subject, while only a magnified detail of the fundus image is shown. The first step was to combine three sequential monochrome frames to one color frame (Fig. 5.7a). In the next step, a white balance was applied to correct different luminosities of the LED emitters. Those differences were constant and were known by a calibration measurement. Within the same step, a gamma correction was applied to enhance the contrast (Fig. 5.7b). In the next step, a reference frame was subtracted to reduce remaining artifacts caused by the optics and the reproducible part of the image noise (Fig. 5.7c). This reference frame was generated once by a calibration measurement, where the subject was replaced by an absorber. This yielded a "dark frame" containing the optical artifacts and the reproducible part of the image noise. To reduce the variable part of the noise, several "dark frames" were acquired and were averaged to one reference image. The steps described so far (except the reference measurement) were performed for every frame of a video sequence.

In the next step, those frames were registered, which means that the frames are shifted so that movements of the fundus were compensated. After that, they were superimposed and averaged to one single image. The effect is a suppression of image content that occurs only at one or a few frames. Thus, the non-reproducible part of the image noise is suppressed (Fig. 5.7d). Finally the clarity was increased by a spatial high-pass filter (Fig. 5.7e). The last two steps (Fig. 5.7d, e) only were possible by the video capability of the device. Figure 5.8 shows the whole post-processed fundus image manually stitched together with two other stripe-field images of different areas of the retina. The size of one stripe is 68° by 18°.

The described image processing procedure is borrowed from amateur astronomy, where videos are made of planets with a video camera [13], while turbulences in the atmosphere are randomly shifting the planet image. The procedure could be adopted very well, because there were

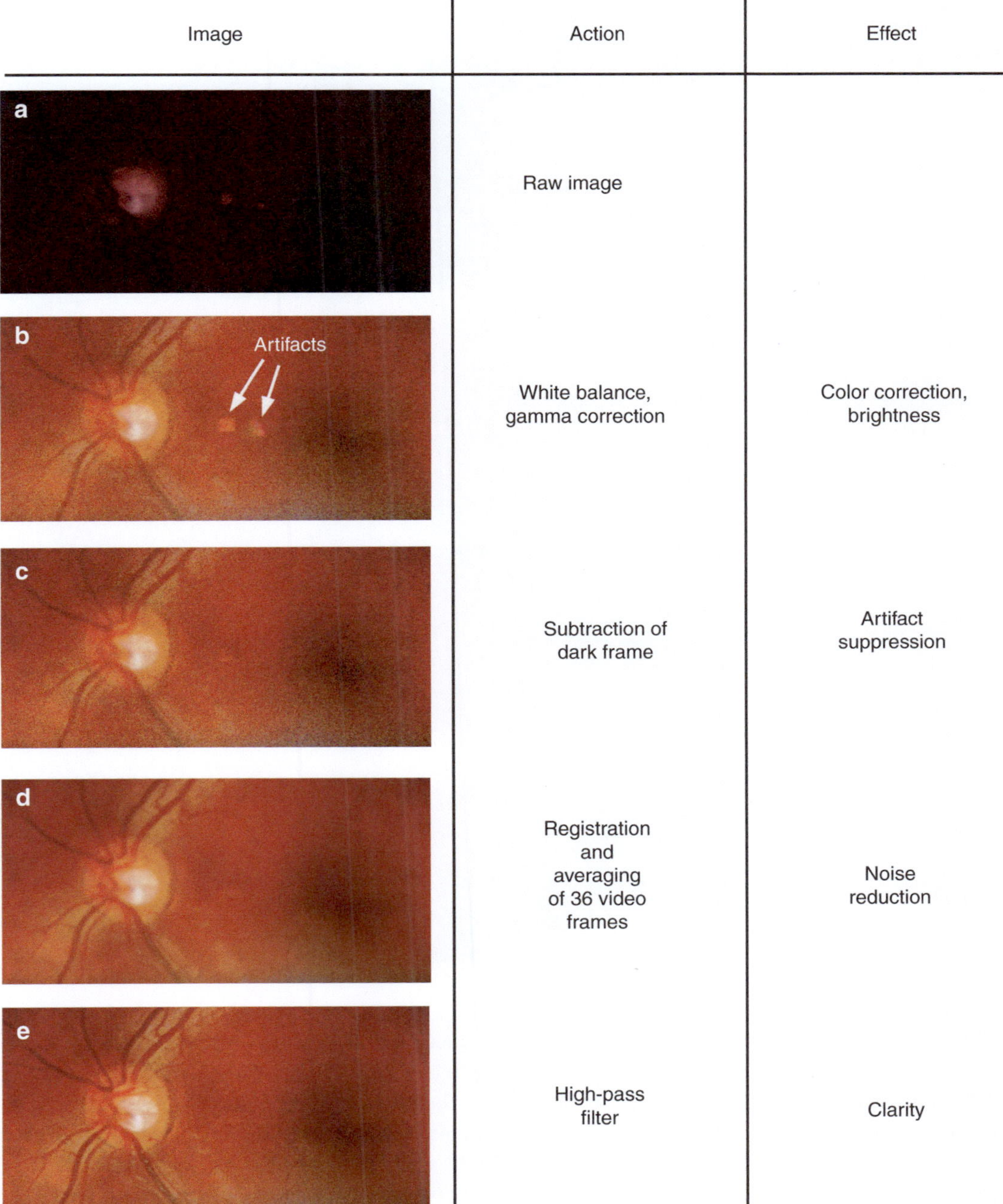

Fig. 5.7 Enhancing the image quality by digital image post-processing taking advantage of the video capability. (**a**) raw image (**b**) gamma correction (**c**) subtraction of dark frame (**d**) registration and averaging (**e**) high pass filter

similar conditions: a non-changing object, which moves randomly, and a noisy image. This is why a software intended for video astronomy called "Giotto" directly could be used to perform registration, averaging, reference frame subtraction, and high-pass filtering.

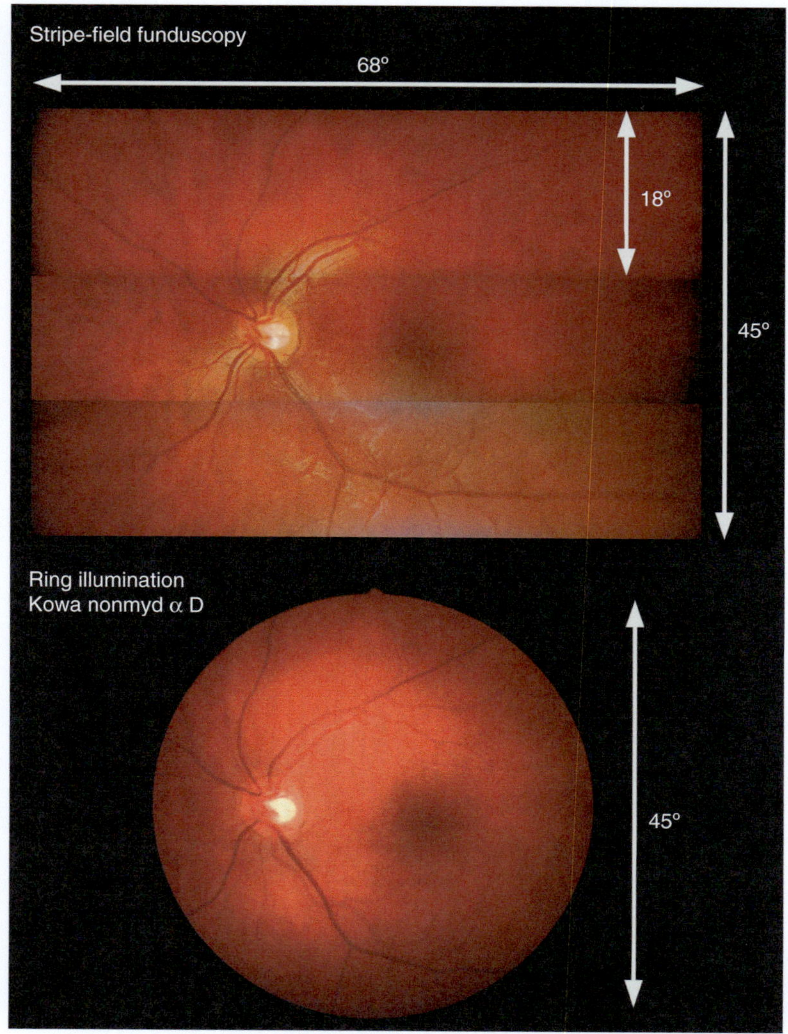

Fig. 5.8 Stitched stripe-field fundus image compared with standard fundus image

5.10 Results

The fundus video camera was tested with 31 healthy subjects with ages reaching from 22 to 52 with an average age of 29.9 years. Refractive errors were present at 52.9 % of the subjects, which did not wear visual aids during the video acquirement. The method could be tested successfully with 27 of the subjects and delivered videos [12] of the fundus. With the remaining four subjects, the method could not be fully tested as the shape of their faces did not allow getting close enough to the eye to reach the optimal working distance of 20 mm. Thus, the field of view was reduced for those four subjects. Using eyepieces with larger working distances, which are available on the market, should solve this problem. The acquired frame rate was four frames per second with an exposure time of 16 ms each. The light energy per frame entering the eye was below 3 μJ, and the average light power was 30 μW.

To demonstrate dynamic effects within the eye, a fundus video was acquired while a 23-year-old healthy subject was slightly touching (Fig. 5.9a) and releasing (Fig. 5.9b) the lid. The resulting video showed changes at vessels in the region of the papilla and a change of the paleness of the papilla.

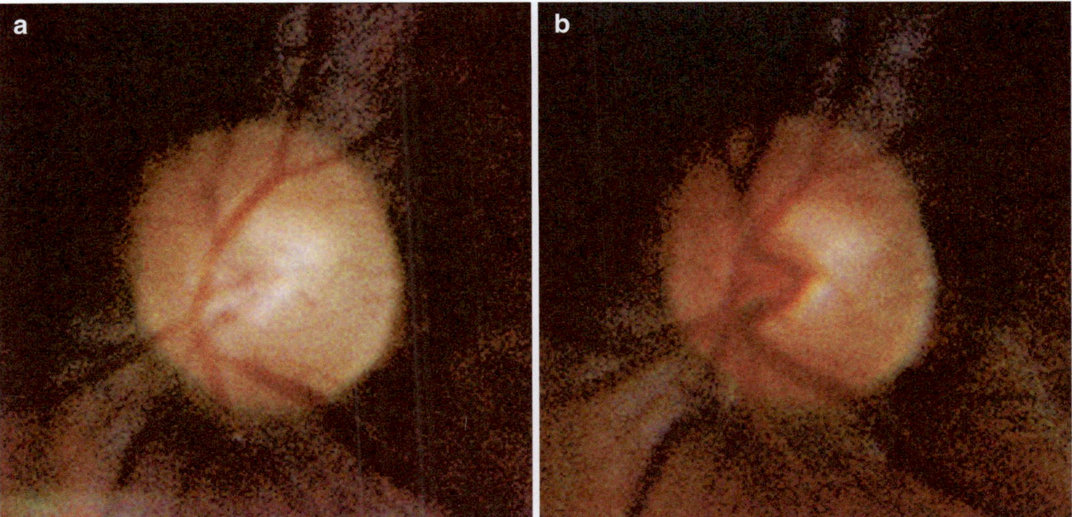

Fig. 5.9 Two frames (detail) of a fundus video showing changes of paleness and vessels at the papilla with (**a**) and without (**b**) external pressure to the eye

5.11   Discussion

The results show that the stripe-field method offers several advantages compared to conventional ring illumination techniques: The field of view at a pupil size of 2 mm could be increased from 314 square degrees (circular area, diameter: 20°) to 1,124 square degrees (rectangular area, 18°×68°), which is nearly a factor of 4. Furthermore, the image repetition rate is not limited in principle enabling the acquisition of video sequences of the fundus. The darkening of examination rooms is not needed any more. The technical outlay of the new method is very low so that a demonstrator could be realized for only about 5,000 US$ compared to 20,000–50,000 US$ for conventional devices. It is nearly a solid-state device as it contains only one movable part. This makes the new design very robust compared to conventional devices. An operation is possible in any orientation; even upside-down usage was demonstrated. A direct comparison of the new design with a conventional device (Kowa Nonmyd α-D) is shown in Fig. 5.8, showing the fundus of the same eye, while the Kowa device operated with 4 mm pupil diameter and the new design with only 2 mm. Finally the new design is lightweight with only

2.9 kg (without the chin rest) compared to 22 kg [14] of the Kowa fundus camera.

All those features make the new stripe-field method very suitable for telemedical applications as it fulfills many requirements being essential for telemedicine: low price, robustness, lightweight, ease of use, high image repetition rate, non-mydriatic, no need for dark examination rooms, video capability, and color operation.

Conclusion

A non-mydriatic color fundus camera was constructed for only 5,000 US$ by using mass-market components. A new imaging method was invented and applied making it possible to capture wide-field color fundus videos or images with 68°×18° field of view at pupil sizes of only 2 mm. The number of moving parts within the camera could be reduced to just one component resulting in a very robust device. Furthermore, an easy way was found to align the camera to the eye, which can be used continuously and parallel to image or video acquisition. By digital post-processing, it was possible to generate a still image from a video with enhanced image clarity. The camera was tested successfully with 27 subjects.

References

1. Everdell NL, Styles IB, Calcagni A, Gibson J, Hebden J, Claridge E. Multispectral imaging of the ocular fundus using light emitting diode illumination. Rev Sci Instrum. 2010;81:093706.
2. Dick M, Mohr T, Bublitz D. Einrichtung und Verfahren zur Beobachtung, Dokumentation und/oder Diagnose des Augenhintergrundes. Patent DE 19626443. 2005.
3. Rassow B, Wesemann W. Moderne Augenrefraktometer. Stuttgart: Ferdinand Enke; 1984.
4. Cornsweet TN, Crane HD. Accurate two-dimensional eye tracker using first and fourth Purkinje images. J Opt Soc Am. 1973;63:8.
5. Helmholtz H. Beschreibung eines Augenspiegels zur Untersuchung der Netzhaut im lebenden Auge. Berlin: A. Förstner'sche Verlagsbuchhandlung; 1851.
6. Ruete TTG. Der Augenspiegel und das Optometer für practische Aerzte. Göttingen: Verlag der Dieterichschen Buchhandlung; 1852.
7. Bublitz D, Müller L, Mohrholz U, Mohr T, Teige F. Fundus camera with strip-shaped pupil division and method for recording artefact-free, high-resolution fundus images. Patent WO 2012/059236. 2011.
8. Pomerantzeff O, Webb RH, Delori FC. Image formation in fundus cameras. Invest Ophthalmol Vis Sci. 1979;18(6):630–7.
9. Heacock GL. Portable fundus viewing system for an undilated eye. Patent US 5861939. 1999.
10. Feldon S, Yoon G. Compact ocular fundus camera. Patent US 7802884. 2010.
11. Tran K, Mendel TA, Holbrook KL, Yates PA. Construction of an inexpensive, hand-held fundus camera through modification of a consumer "point & shoot" camera. Invest Ophthalmol Vis Sci. 2012;53(12):7600–7.
12. Höher B, Voigtmann P, Michelson G, Schmauss B. Non-mydriatic, wide field, fundus video camera. In: Manns F, Söderberg PG, Ho A, editors. Proceedings of the SPIE Photonics West, 1–6 Feb 2014. San Francisco: SPIE; 2014. p. 89300K.
13. Martin A, Koch B. Digitale Astrofotografie: Grundlagen und Praxis der CCD- und Digitalkameratechnik. Erlangen: Oculum; 2009.
14. Kowa Optimed Europe Ltd. Specification sheet of product "Kowa nonmyd-α D" [Internet]. 2014. Available from: http://www.kowa.eu/medicals/en/nonmydaD.php.

Noninvasive Ocular Angiography by Optical Coherence Tomography

6

Yali Jia and David Huang

Contents

Y. Jia, PhD • D. Huang, MD, PhD (✉)
Casey Eye Institute, Oregon Health & Science University, 3375 S.W. Terwilliger Blvd., Portland, OR 97239-4197, USA
e-mail: jiaya@ohsu.edu; huangd@ohsu.edu

6.1　Introduction

The leading causes of blindness such as diabetic retinopathy [1], age-related macular degeneration [2], and glaucoma [3] are all associated with impaired circulation. Examination of ocular circulation is critical for the assessment of these eye diseases. Therefore, noninvasive ocular angiography would be a powerful methodology for understanding and diagnosing these eye diseases.

Currently, the most widely used technique for examining ocular circulation abnormalities is fundus fluorescein angiography (FA). This is an invasive procedure. It requires dye injection which might cause nausea and anaphylaxis. In addition, FA cannot distinguish choroidal vessels from retinal vessels or detect the lamina cribrosa perfusion deep inside the optic nerve head (ONH). Other existing noninvasive imaging techniques, such as scanning laser Doppler flowmetry and scanning laser speckle flowmetry, are also limited to 2D imaging of the superficial perfusion [3].

Optical coherence tomography (OCT) generates cross-sectional images by measuring the echo time delay and magnitude of backscattered light [4]. It has achieved micrometer-level axial resolution in cross-sectional retinal imaging. Currently OCT has been a necessary part of the standard of care for retinal diseases and increasingly so for glaucoma and anterior segment surgeries as well. However, conventional structural OCT cannot provide the blood flow information directly. Doppler OCT has been used to obtain precise measurements

G. Michelson (ed.), *Teleophthalmology in Preventive Medicine*,
DOI 10.1007/978-3-662-44975-2_6, © Springer-Verlag Berlin Heidelberg 2015

of total retinal blood flow calculated from the Doppler frequency shift of backscattered light [5]. While appropriate for large vessels around the disc, Doppler OCT is not sensitive enough to accurately measure the low velocities of small vessels.

We have recently developed a new 3D ocular angiography using optical coherence tomography (OCT). The algorithm is called split-spectrum amplitude-decorrelation angiography (SSADA) [6]. By splitting the full OCT spectrum into several narrower bands, SSADA reduces OCT axial resolution and consequently reduces its susceptibility to axial motion noise. These changes enable improved detection of the flow signal, which in the ocular fundus is predominantly in the transverse dimension. With a ~3 s scan using our 100 kHz swept-source OCT prototype, SSADA provides a high-quality $3 \times 3 \times 3$ mm 3D angiogram. By selecting the maximum value along the axial (Z) direction or by slicing the angiographic volume at each layer, 3D OCT angiography can produce different types of X-Y projection angiograms for retinal, choroidal, and ONH circulation. In the following sections, the system and theory of OCT angiography and its performance will be demonstrated.

6.2   System and Scan Pattern

Our OCT angiography studies use a high-speed swept-source OCT system recently developed by our group at the Massachusetts Institute of Technology [7] for 3D *in vivo* imaging of the human eye. To enhance the choroidal penetration and increase imaging depth, we use a swept light source with a central wavelength of 1,050 nm. The laser sweep range is 100 nm, providing an axial resolution of 5.3 µm (full-width-half-maximum amplitude profile) and a total depth range of 2.9 mm in the tissue. The laser sweep has a repetition rate of 100 kHz. The emitted light from the laser is split into the sample and reference arms. In the sample arm, a focused spot of 18 µm diameter (full-width-half-maximum amplitude profile) is achieved on the retinal plane. The light returning from the reference and sample arms interferes and is detected by a balanced receiver.

The scanning protocol has been optimized to implement the SSADA. For example, in the fast

transverse scan (X) direction, the B-scan contains 200 A-lines covering 3 mm. With this configuration, the B-scan frame rate of the system is 455 frames per second. In the slow transverse scan (Y) direction, 200 sampling positions covering 3 mm are used to capture a 3D data set, with eight repeated B-scans at every position. The eight repeated B-frames (M-B-frames) are used for the SSADA calculation to obtain both the structure and blood flow images. Therefore, 1,600 B-scans are acquired to form a 3D data cube within an acquisition time of 3.5 s.

6.3   Split-Spectrum Amplitude-Decorrelation Angiography (SSADA) Algorithm

The speckle decorrelation phenomenon is clearly observed in real-time OCT reflectance images where the scattering pattern of blood flow varies rapidly over time due to the flow stream that drives randomly distributed blood cells through the imaging volume. It results in decorrelation of the received backscattered signals that are a function of scatterer displacement over time, creating a contrast between decorrelated blood flow and nondecorrelated static tissue that can be used to extract flow signals for angiography.

In contrast to Doppler and other phase-based approaches in Fourier-domain OCT, amplitude-decorrelation measurement is sensitive to transverse flow and immune to phase noise. However, the high axial resolution of swept-source OCT makes it very sensitive to the pulsatile bulk eye motion noise in the axial direction. In the fundus, ocular pulsation mainly occurs along the axial direction and is driven by the retrobulbar orbital tissue in relation to the heartbeat. The high sensitivity in that direction results in unacceptable signal-to-noise ratio (SNR). To overcome this limitation, we created the SSADA algorithm based on the decorrelation of OCT signal amplitude due to flow.

The basic procedures of SSADA are shown in Fig. 6.1. The high-resolution OCT amplitude frames (M-B-frames) transformed by the full spectrum are not used for amplitude-decorrelation computation. The key step of SSADA (Figs. 6.1 and 6.2) is splitting the raw full spectrum into multiple spectrums with

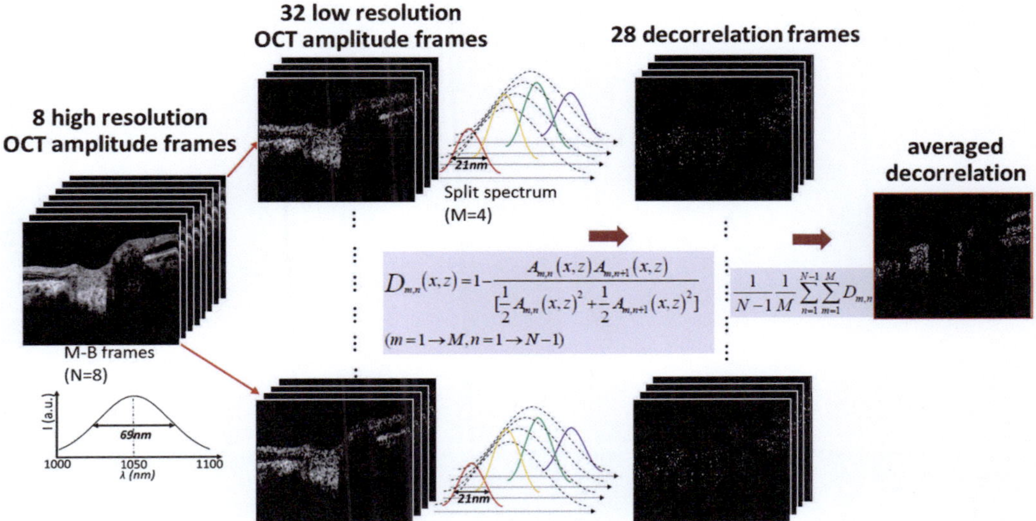

$$D_{m,n}(x,z) = 1 - \frac{A_{m,n}(x,z)\,A_{m,n+1}(x,z)}{[\frac{1}{2}A_{m,n}(x,z)^2 + \frac{1}{2}A_{m,n+1}(x,z)^2]}$$

$$(m = 1 \rightarrow M, n = 1 \rightarrow N-1)$$

$$\frac{1}{N-1}\frac{1}{M}\sum_{n=1}^{N-1}\sum_{m=1}^{M}D_{m,n}$$

Fig. 6.1 Flow chart detailing the basic steps of the split-spectrum amplitude-decorrelation angiography (SSADA) algorithm. Eight optical coherence tomography (OCT) repeated B-frames (M-B-frames) were scanned consecutively at the same spatial location to produce 8 spectral interferograms and 8 standard-resolution cross-sectional images. Using SSADA, each full spectral interferogram was split into 4 spectral bands creating 32 low-resolution interferograms. B-scan decorrelation of each split band yielded 28 decorrelation frames which were averaged to produce one final decorrelation-based flow cross section with improved quality

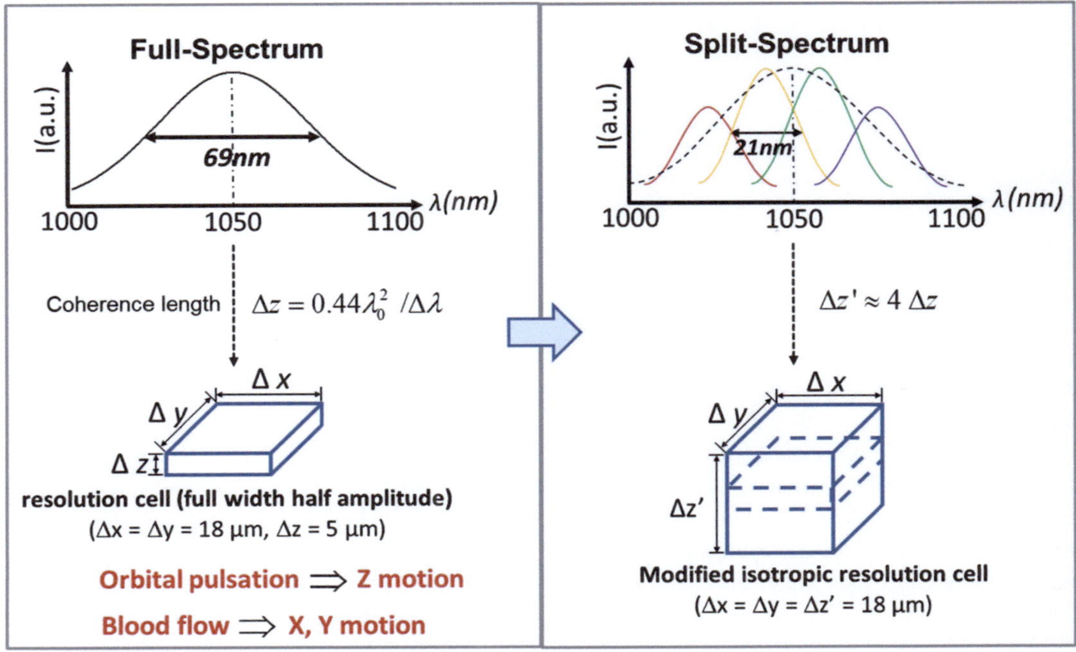

Fig. 6.2 Diagram of the modification of the optical coherence tomography (OCT) imaging resolution cell using the split-spectrum method. The resolution cell ($x = y > z$) in the current configuration can be modified into a new resolution cell ($x = y = z'$)

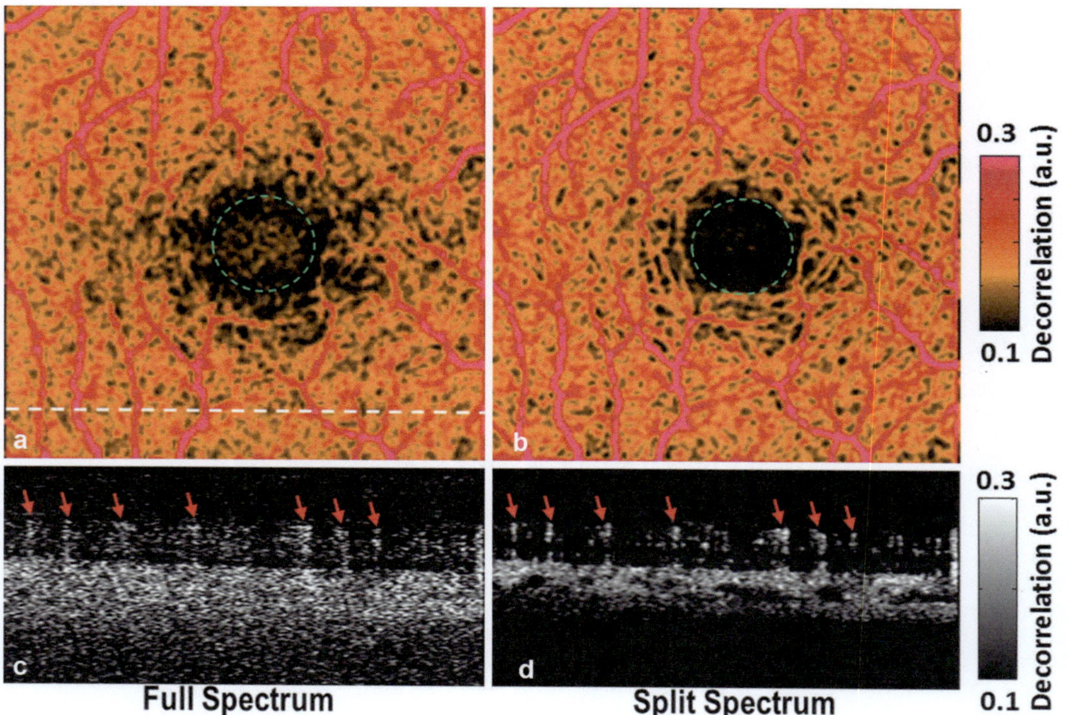

Fig. 6.3 Comparison of amplitude-decorrelation angiograms of the macula (3×3 mm area) using full-spectrum (**a**, **c**) and split-spectrum (**b**, **d**) algorithms. Three-dimensional (3D) angiography scans were acquired on a 100 kHz optical coherence tomography (OCT) prototype. With the novel split-spectrum algorithm, *en face* maximum decorrelation projections of the retinal circulation showed less noise inside the foveal avascular zone (FAZ, inside *green dotted circles*) and a more continuous perifoveal vascular network using the novel split-spectrum algorithm (**b**) compared to the standard full-spectrum algorithm (**a**). The signal-to-noise ratio (SNR), computed by dividing the perifoveal flow signal by the false flow signal in the FAZ, is 2.1 times higher using the split-spectrum algorithm [6]. The cross-sectional angiograms (scanned across the *red dashed line* in **a**) showed more clearly delineated retinal vessels (*red arrows*) and choroidal layers and less noise using the split-spectrum algorithm (**d**) compared to the standard full-spectrum algorithm (**c**)

narrow bandwidths. Narrower bandwidth is intentionally created to lower the OCT axial resolution. This minimizes the noise along the axial direction and optimizes flow detection along the transverse direction (Fig. 6.2). After the narrower spectra are Fourier transformed, low-resolution OCT amplitude frames are used to calculate decorrelation. Inter-B-scan decorrelation can be determined at each of the narrower spectral bands separately and then averaged. Recombining the decorrelation images from the multiple narrow spectral bands yields angiograms that use the full information in the entire OCT spectral range. The recent work [6] shows that such images (Fig. 6.3b, d) produce significant improve-

ment of SNR for both flow detection and connectivity of microvascular networks when compared to full-spectrum amplitude-decorrelation techniques (Fig. 6.3a, c).

Furthermore, the full OCT spectrum is split into several narrower spectral bands, resulting in an OCT resolution cell in each band which is isotropic and less susceptible to axial motion noise (Fig. 6.2). Creation of isotropic resolution cells having equal sensitivity to axial and transverse flow can be useful for quantifying flow. In other words, OCT angiography extracts flow information that can be further processed for quantification because the flow values generated by the isotropic resolution cells are a function of the flow velocity regardless of direction.

6.4 Retinal and Choroidal Circulation

The macular region of the fundus is responsible for central vision. Capillary dropout in the macular region due to diabetic retinopathy is a major cause of vision loss. Focal loss of the choriocapillaris is a possible causative factor in the pathogenesis of both dry and wet age-related macular degeneration [8], the leading cause of blindness in industrialized countries [9]. Thus, macular angiography is important.

The SSADA is used to demonstrate macular angiography of both the retinal and choroidal circulations in a normal eye (Fig. 6.4). The 3D SSADA data set comprises a stack of 200 averaged decorrelation cross-sectional images, along with the associated averaged reflectance images, that span 3 mm in the slow transverse scan (Y) direction (Fig. 6.4a). The 3D data is separated into retinal and choroidal regions with the dividing boundary set at the retinal pigment epithelium (RPE) (see yellow line in Fig. 6.4). The

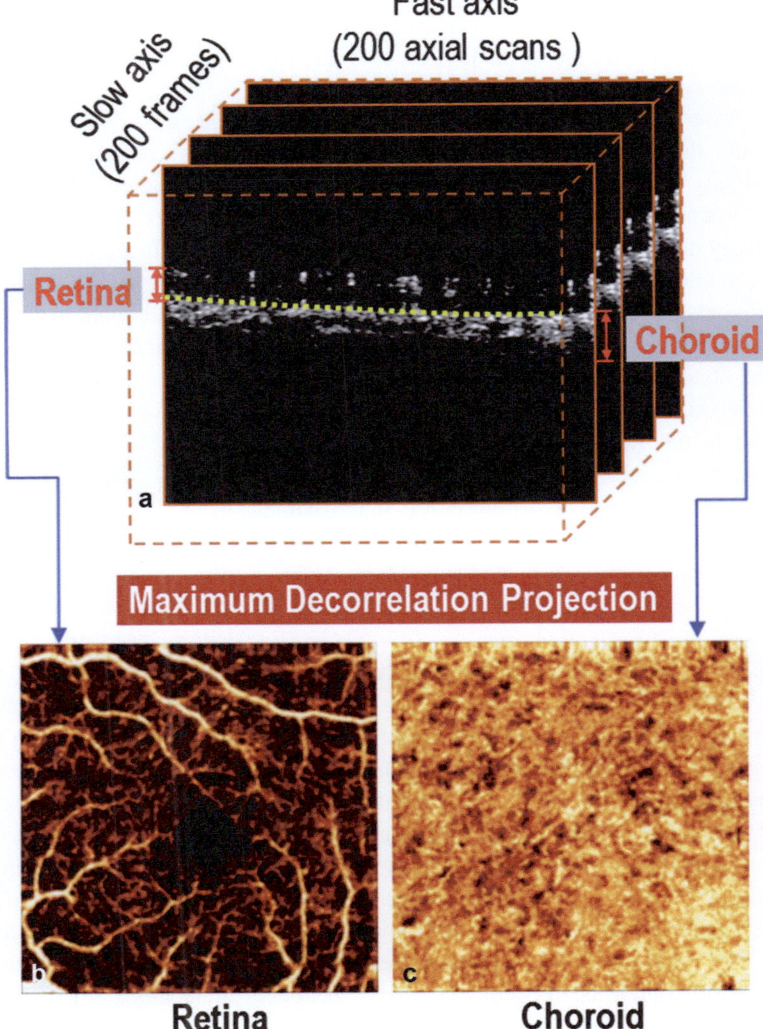

Fig. 6.4 Segmentation and processing of an optical coherence tomography (OCT) angiogram of a normal macula. (**a**) The 3D OCT angiogram comprises 200 frames of averaged decorrelation cross sections stretched along the slow scan axis. Each frame is computed using the split-spectrum amplitude-decorrelation angiography (SSADA) algorithm shown in Fig. 6.1. The angiogram spans 3 mm in all 3 dimensions. The cross-sectional angiogram shows the retinal and choroidal circulations along the retinal pigment epithelium (RPE) boundary (*dotted yellow line*). The retina and choroid were separately projected. (**b**) The retina angiogram shows the retinal vessels become smaller toward the fovea ending in parafoveal capillary net with no flow detected in the foveal avascular zone (FAZ). (**c**) The choroidal angiogram shows a near-confluent high-flow network

depth (Z direction) of the highly reflective RPE is identified through the analysis of the reflectance and reflectance gradient profiles [10]. The region above the RPE is the retinal layer, and the region below is the choroidal layer. The *en face* X-Y projection angiograms (Fig. 6.4b, c) are produced by selecting the maximum decorrelation value along the axial (Z) direction in each layer.

The flow pixels form a continuous microcirculatory network in the retina. The vascular network is absent in the foveal avascular zone (Fig. 6.4b) of approximately 600 μm diameter, in agreement with known anatomy. There are some disconnected apparent flow pixels within the foveal avascular zone (Fig. 6.4b) due to noise. The choriocapillaris layer forms a confluent overlapping plexus [11], so it is to be expected that the projection image of the choroidal circulation shows confluent flow (Fig. 6.4c).

Based on the decorrelation seen in the gray scale, the flow in the inner choroid has higher velocity. The volume is also greater than the retinal circulation, again consistent with known physiology that the choroidal circulation has much higher flow than the retinal circulation [11]. There are signal voids in the outer choroid that may be due to fringe washout from high flow velocity and the shadowing effect of overlying tissue. The cross sections also show a few spots of decorrelation in the RPE layer. These must be artifacts because the RPE is avascular. This is likely due to the projection of flow decorrelation in a proximal layer (i.e., inner retinal layers) onto distal layers which have a strong reflected signal (i.e., RPE).

6.5 Optic Nerve Head Circulation

Circumstantial evidence suggests that ONH ischemia may be a causative factor for optic neuropathy disease such as glaucoma, the leading cause of blindness in the USA. ONH perfusion may also correlate with the pathogenesis of multiple sclerosis with optic neuritis. Thus, the ONH angiogram is also very important.

The SSADA is used to demonstrate ONH angiography in a normal eye (Fig. 6.5). Cross-sectional SSADA angiograms (Fig. 6.5a) show both large and small vessels in the retina, choroid, and ONH. The microvascular network is nearly confluent in the choriocapillaris, very dense in the ONH, and sparser in the retina. The normal ONH angiogram shows dense vasculature from the prelaminar tissue to the deep lamina cribrosa in the choroidal and scleral planes (Fig. 6.5a). As mentioned in the last section, a limitation of OCT angiography is the "projection" artifact, where the transit of blood cells in a superficial blood vessel cast flickering shadows on the deeper tissue layer, which is indistinguishable from flow. Examples of the projection artifact can also be seen in the cross-sectional ONH angiogram (Fig. 6.5a), where flow in the superficial retinal vessels is projected onto deeper retinal layers, including the avascular pigment epithelium. The projection artifact is less problematic when the 3D SSADA angiogram is summarized and viewed as *en face* maximum decorrelation projections. The projection process can separate ONH, retinal, and choroidal circulations along 3D anatomic division planes (Fig. 6.5b, c). Unlike scanning laser techniques (laser Doppler flowmetry and laser speckle flowgraphy), OCT angiography can image the deep ONH circulation (lamina cribrosa) as well as more superficial disc and retinal vessels [12].

6.6 Large View of Ocular Angiography

To achieve a clinically applicable imaging method, the capability to image a large field of view is critical. However, the scanning patterns and the acquisition speed presented in this study do not allow for larger than the 3×3 mm scanning area. This was because of the need to maintain high-resolution with acquisition time in a single volume of a few seconds. To overcome this limitation, we acquired several volumes centered at different retinal locations. Figure 6.6 shows an example of the large field of view image. This image was made from twelve 3×3 mm OCT angiography volumes acquired by shifting the position of fixation points. Processed by SSADA, each projection image was manually aligned with linear translation to create a large field of view mosaic.

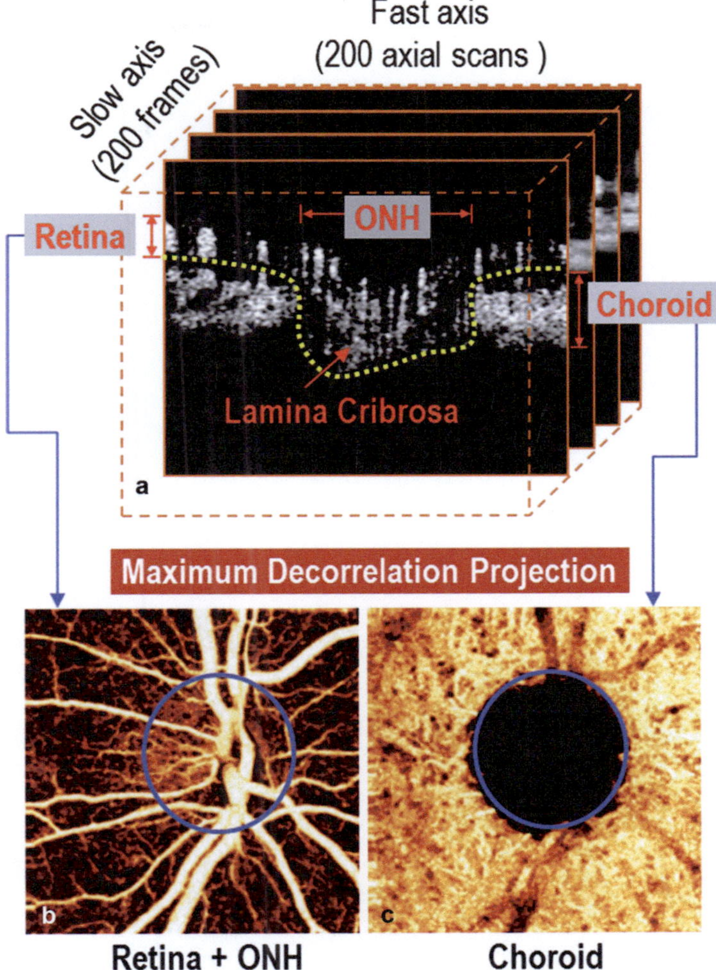

Fig. 6.5 Segmentation and processing of an optical coherence tomography (OCT) angiogram of a normal optic nerve head (ONH). (**a**) The 3D OCT angiogram comprises 200 frames of averaged decorrelation cross sections stretched along the slow scan axis. Each frame is computed using the split-spectrum amplitude-decorrelation angiography (SSADA) algorithm shown in Fig. 6.1. The angiogram spans 3 mm in all 3 dimensions. The cross-sectional angiogram shows dense ONH microcirculation from the disc surface to the lamina cribrosa. Image processing software separates the retinal and choroidal circulations along the retinal pigment epithelium (RPE) boundary (*dotted yellow line*). The ONH region is lumped with the retinal layers and projected onto a retina + ONH *en face* angiogram. The choroid is separately projected. (**b**) The retina + ONH angiogram shows both large retinal vessels and a microvascular network that is very dense within the ONH and sparser outside. (**c**) The choroidal angiogram shows a near-confluent high-flow network and shadows cast by overlying large retinal vessels. The disc margin is indicated by *blue circle* in **b** and **c**

6.7 Summary

We developed a novel optical angiography technique—SSADA—that can be used to noninvasively visualize the vasculature and blood flow in the posterior eye. This technique is based on the decorrelation of OCT signal amplitude due to blood flow. By splitting the full OCT spectral interferogram into several narrow spectral bands, the OCT resolution cell in each band is less susceptible to axial motion noise. Recombining the decorrelation images from the spectral bands

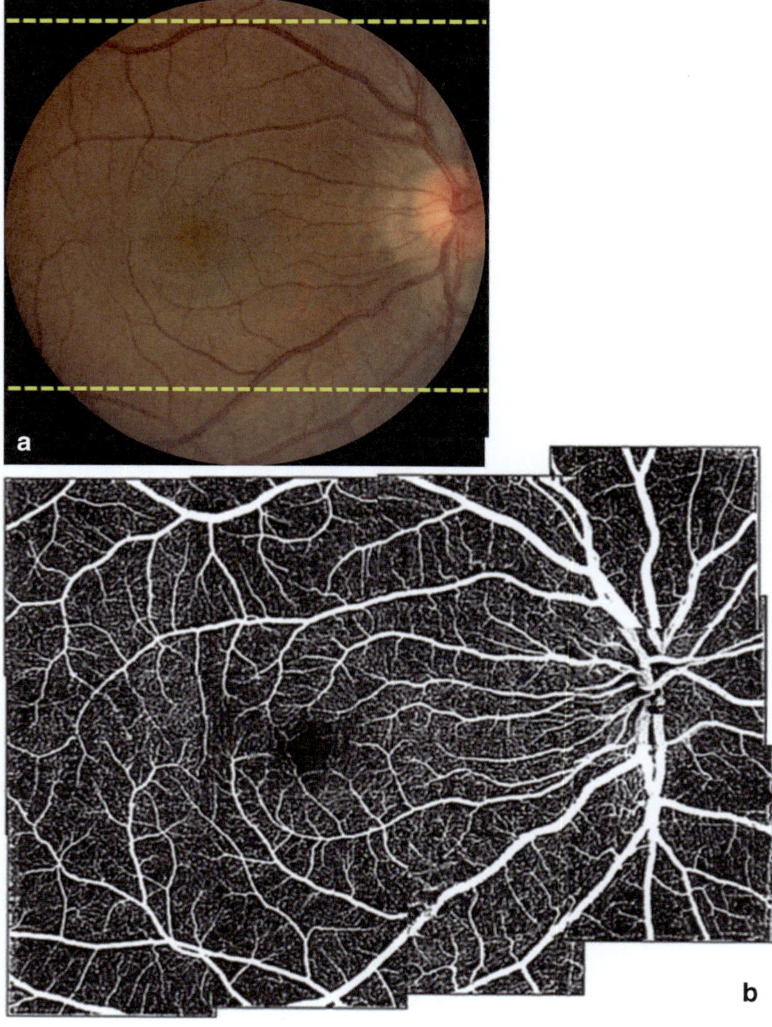

Fig. 6.6 (**a**) Fundus photograph. (**b**) Large field of view stitched optical coherence tomography (OCT) angiography with 12 volumes. Total image acquisition time for 12 volumetric images is approximately 40 s

yields angiograms that use the full information in the entire OCT spectral range.

Besides its noninvasive nature, OCT angiography has several compelling characteristics that make it a promising modality for clinical use. OCT angiography can be acquired in a few seconds, compared to several minutes for FA. Its 3D imaging allows for depth resolution of pathology and separation of individual vascular layers for evaluation. Quantitative information, such as vessel density, vessel area, and flow index, can now be obtained. The OCT angiography scan pattern and SSADA processing can be implemented on

spectral-domain or swept-source OCT systems without any special hardware modification.

There are several limitations to OCT angiography. High speed is needed to provide sufficient cross-sectional frame rate to overcome background eye motion. Therefore, the current generation of commercial OCT systems at 20–40 kHz speed may be insufficient. The next generation of OCT system running at 70–100 kHz is likely required. In the present study, the 100 kHz OCT prototype image provided a small 3 mm square field of view. We have recently improved the scan and processing software to provide a 4 mm field of view. However, even larger field of view will require even higher speed. Because laboratory OCT prototypes of multi-MHz speed have already been reported [13–15], we believe the speed and scan size area limitations will be solved as commercial implementation catches up to laboratory technology. Finally, OCT angiography does not identify leakage and staining on FA. But OCT can provide other markers, such as intraretinal cysts, retinal thickening, subretinal fluid, and angiographic flow index.

Overall, OCT angiography is faster and more sensitive and has deeper depth penetration than other angiography modalities. It is a promising new method for comprehensive investigation of blood flow in the eye.

References

1. Patel V, Rassam S, Newsom R, Wiek J, Kohner E. Retinal blood flow in diabetic retinopathy. BMJ. 1992;305(6855):678–83. 1992-09-19 00:00:00.
2. Friedman E. A hemodynamic model of the pathogenesis of age-related macular degeneration. Am J Ophthalmol. 1997;124(5):677–82.
3. Flammer J, Orgül S, Costa VP, Orzalesi N, Krieglstein GK, Serra LM, et al. The impact of ocular blood flow in glaucoma. Prog Retin Eye Res. 2002;21(4):359–93.
4. Huang D, Swanson EA, Lin CP, Schuman JS, Stinson WG, Chang W, et al. Optical coherence tomography. Science (New York, NY). 1991;254(5035):1178–81.
5. Wang Y, Bower BA, Izatt JA, Tan O, Huang D. Retinal blood flow measurement by circumpapillary Fourier domain Doppler optical coherence tomography. J Biomed Opt. 2008;13(6):064003.
6. Jia Y, Tan O, Tokayer J, Potsaid B, Wang Y, Liu JJ, et al. Split-spectrum amplitude-decorrelation angiography with optical coherence tomography. Opt Express. 2012;20(4):4710–25.
7. Potsaid B, Baumann B, Huang D, Barry S, Cable AE, Schuman JS, et al. Ultrahigh speed 1050 nm swept source/Fourier domain OCT retinal and anterior segment imaging at 100,000 to 400,000 axial scans per second. Opt Express. 2010;18(19):20029–48.
8. Zhao J, Frambach DA, Lee PP, Lee M, Lopez PF. Delayed macular choriocapillary circulation in age-related macular degeneration. Int Ophthalmol. 1995;19(1):1–12.
9. Bressler NM. Age-related macular degeneration is the leading cause of blindness. JAMA. 2004;291(15):1900–1.
10. An L, Wang RK. In vivo volumetric imaging of vascular perfusion within human retina and choroids with optical micro-angiography. Opt Express. 2008;16(15):11438–52.
11. Roh S, Weiter JJ. Retinal and choroidal circulation. In: Yanoff M, Duker JS, editors. Ophthalmology. St. Louis: Mosby Elsevier; 2008.
12. Jia Y, Morrison JC, Tokayer J, Tan O, Lombardi L, Baumann B, et al. Quantitative OCT angiography of optic nerve head blood flow. Biomed Opt Express. 2012;3(12):3127.
13. Choi D-h, Hiro-Oka H, Shimizu K, Ohbayashi K. Spectral domain optical coherence tomography of multi-MHz A-scan rates at 1310 nm range and real-time 4D-display up to 41 volumes/second. Biomed Opt Express. 2012;3(12):3067–86.
14. Klein T, Wieser W, André R, Pfeiffer T, Eigenwillig CM, Huber R. Multi-MHz FDML OCT: snapshot retinal imaging at 6.7 million axial-scans per second. Proceeding of SPIE 8213; 2012 Feb 2–11; San Francisco. Bellingham: Publisher SPIE; 2012. p. 82131E.
15. Potsaid B, Jayaraman V, Fujimoto JG, Jiang J, Heim PJS, Cable AE. MEMS tunable VCSEL light source for ultrahigh speed 60 kHz–1 MHz axial scan rate and long range centimeter class OCT imaging. Proceeding of SPIE 8213; 2012 Feb 2–11; San Francisco. Bellingham: Publisher SPIE; 2012. p. 82130M.

Adaptive Optics Imaging of the Retina and Vessels

7

Michel Paques

Contents

Adaptive optics (AO) is an optoelectronic technique that allows counteracting the optical aberrations generated by the anterior segment by means of a deformable mirror. AO allows increasing the lateral (not the axial) resolution of fundus images down to the micrometric scale. An increasing number of clinical applications are identified for AO imaging; hence, it is progressively translating from the lab to the clinics and will undoubtedly become a routine procedure for many retinal diseases in the next years. AO reflectance imaging has been implemented in two configurations of fundus imaging technology: flood imaging and confocal scanning laser ophthalmoscopy. These techniques yield somewhat different results; this presentation will deal only with flood imaging AO.

Although AO fundus imaging technology is reaching technological maturity, clinical interpretation of the complex features of diseased retina remains challenging. The first photoreceptor images using AO were obtained more than 15 years ago [1] However, integration of AO images in the diagnostic process has not been as straightforward as for optical coherence tomography; AO images are indeed sometimes challenging to interpret because a number of factors may interfere in the images obtained from a diseased retina. Among these factors are the level of pigmentation of the fundus, the transparency of the retina itself (any loss of transparency of the inner retina will disperse light and hence blur the images of photoreceptors), the presence of other sources of light reflection in diseased retina, the

M. Paques, MD, PhD
Clinical Investigation Center 1423,
Quinze-Vingts Hospital, University Pierre
et Marie Curie-Paris6, Paris, France
e-mail: mp@cicoph.org

G. Michelson (ed.), *Teleophthalmology in Preventive Medicine*,
DOI 10.1007/978-3-662-44975-2_7, © Springer-Verlag Berlin Heidelberg 2015

spaital, functional and temporal variability of photoreceptor reflectance, and the variable pointing of photoreceptor outer segments. Nevertheless, we will show here some clinical applications of AO in public health diseases that already offer promising opportunities for clinicians. We focused our interest on geographic atrophy, hypertensive retinopathy, and diabetic retinopathy.

7.1   Methods

En face AO fundus images were obtained using an AO retinal camera (rtx1; Imagine Eyes, Orsay, France). The rtx1 camera probes wavefront aberrations with a 750 nm super luminescent diode and a Shack-Hartmann detector (HASO 32-eye; Imagine Eyes) and corrects them with a 52 actuators AO system operating in a closed loop. The fundus is illuminated with a temporally low-coherence light-emitting diode flashed flood source operating at 840 nm. The resolving power claimed by the rtx1 manufacturer (Imagine Eyes) is 250 line pairs per millimeter; this corresponds to a lateral resolution comprised between 2 and 4 μm. In the z-axis, the theoretical focus depth is 52 μm for a 5 mm pupil size and 35.7 μm for a 6 mm pupil. Clinically, its depth of field is small enough to allow focusing on at least two levels in the healthy retina (i.e., vessels or photoreceptor).

Pharmacologic pupil dilation using tropicamide (Mydriaticum; Novartis, France) was done in cases where the pupil size was smaller than 4 mm. The imaging procedure is briefly summarized thereafter: the patient placed their head on a standard ophthalmic chin rest and was instructed to look at an internal fixation target, which is manually oriented by the operator to capture the region of interest (ROI). Focus was done at the cone photoreceptor layer by displacing a cursor in the software graphic user interface while watching the live retinal image displayed by the monitor. Once the ROI has been detected and the focus adjusted, a stack of fundus images are acquired at a rate of 9.5 frames per second over 4.2 s in a 4°×4° area by a charge-coupled device camera (Roper Scientific, Tucson, AZ). It

is estimated that in emmetropic eyes each image covers a 1.2×1.2 mm area. One or two images could be acquired per minute.

7.2   Image Processing

After each acquisition, the resulting series of 40 images was automatically processed by the system's software (A0image 2.0) as follows: the 20 images that presented the best contrast were automatically selected based on their average Sobel contrast. The Sobel contrast sum was computed by applying a classical Sobel filter to each image and averaging the absolute pixel values of the resulting filtered image. The 20 selected images were registered together using an algorithm based on autocorrelation and then added together in order to obtain a summed image with improved signal-to-noise ratio. A background image was computed by applying a Gaussian filter to the summed image. The SD of the Gaussian filter was 25 pixels. The background image was then subtracted from the summed image in order to facilitate the visualization of small details. The brightness and contrast of the resulting image were optimized by stretching the normalized histogram in order to cover the range from 0 to 1 while saturating the brightest pixels in the image. The number of saturated pixels was set to 0.05 % of the total pixel number. Finally, the image was oversampled with a ratio of 1:2 using bicubic interpolation. For morphometric measures of retinal vessels, a dedicated software (AOV, designed by Florence Rossant, ISEP, France) has been used. Time-lapse images were constructed using Adobe Photoshop (Fig. 7.1).

7.3   Results

7.3.1   AO Imaging of Drusens and Geographic Atrophy

We examined patients with variable severity of GA. Drusens appeared as hyperreflective, round- or doughnut-shaped lesions with often a hyporeflective center. The photoreceptor mosaic remains visible over the drusen in most cases (Fig. 7.2).

In areas of GA, as compared to scanning laser ophthalmoscope imaging, AO NIR imaging dramatically improved the resolution of the limits of atrophic areas as well as the redistribution of melanin-loaded cells (Fig. 7.3). A striking feature was indeed the presence of multiple hyporeflective clumps within and around GA areas, which gave a "salt and pepper" appearance to the posterior pole [2]. Of particular interest are the cases with foveal sparing, for which AO can give a very precise delineation of the central island of preserved RPE cells (Fig. 7.4).

We also investigated by time-lapse imaging the kinetics of the progression of atrophy and of pigment redistribution. Successive AO images taken several weeks apart were registered, which allowed the observation of the emergence and progression of atrophic spots. Time-lapse observation also showed the dynamic aspect of the redistribution of melanin-loaded cells such dynamic changes were observed within as well as outside atrophic areas. While limited changes were noted in some cases, many showed a more complex figure, with appearance of new clumps, change in their size and/or shape, rearrangement of large melanin deposits or abrupt disappearance.

7.3.2 AO Imaging of Retinal Vessels

Arterial hypertension, diabetes, and age affect the structure of retinal vessels. An increase of the wall-to-lumen ratio (WLR) of small arteries is a

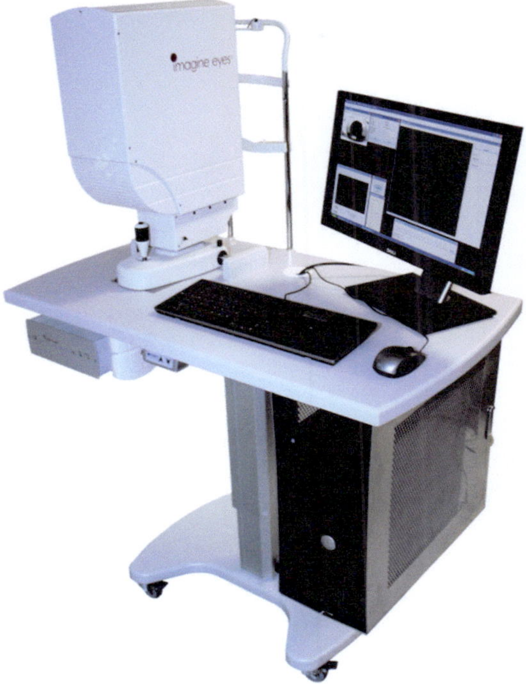

Fig. 7.1 Flood imaging adaptive optics funds camera developed by Imagine Eyes

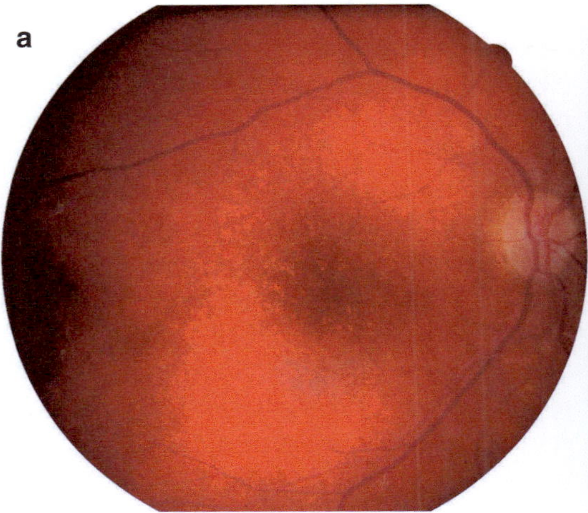
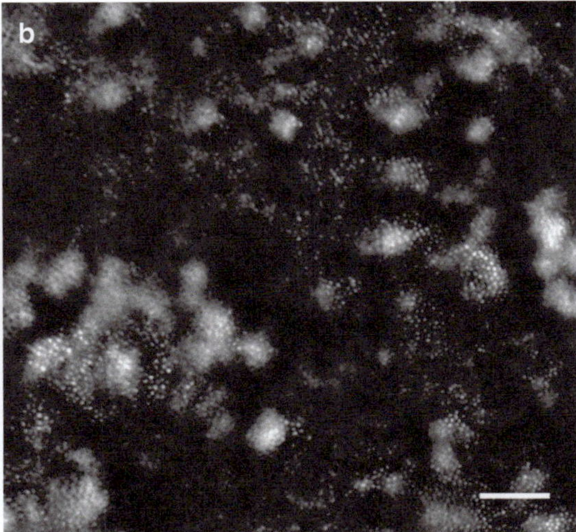

Fig. 7.2 Typical aspect of drusens by AO imaging. (**a**) *Left*, color photograph; (**b**) *right*, AO image of the area indicated in the *square* (bar, 100 μm)

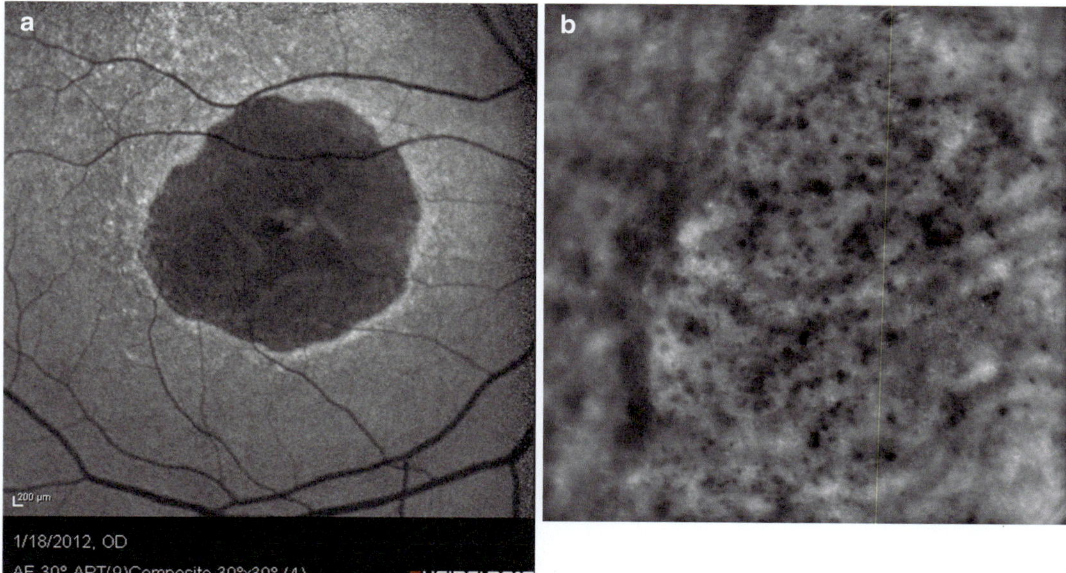

Fig. 7.3 Case of geographic atrophy. (**a**) *Left*, 488 nm autofluorescence image; (**b**) *right*, AO image of the area indicated in square. Note the better resolution of the limits of the GA area as well as the observation of a myriad of melanin clumps (bar, 250 μm)

hallmark of hypertensive microangiopathy and is predictive of end-organ damage such as stroke [3]. Using conventional fundus photographs, several large-scale epidemiological studies reported that arteriolar narrowing and the incidence of focal arteriolar narrowing (FAN) and arteriovenous nicking (AVN) correlates with past and incident arterial pressure and with end-organ damage such as coronary diseases [4, 5] and stroke [6]. The clinical evaluation of hypertensive retinopathy is however impaired by technical limitations, mostly because fundus photographs or fluorescein angiography do not enable visualizing the arteriolar wall.

By AO NIR imaging, a linear structure is visible along both sides of the blood column of arteries (Fig. 7.5). In order to extract morphometric parameters from these images, we designed a software to automatically segment parietal structures (only images taken in diastole were considered for such analysis in order to minimize motion blur). The ratio of total parietal thickness over the lumen diameter (D) defined the WLR. This parameter was measured in the superotemporal artery in a cohort of 49 treatment-naïve patients [7]. In multivariate analysis taking into account age, gender, lumen diameter, body mass index, and systolic, diastolic, mean, and pulse blood pressure, only mean blood pressure and lumen diameter were independently correlated to WLR, which is in agreement with the concept that a myogenic reflex accounts for parietal thickening [8].

While it is commonly assumed that diffuse parietal thickening is initiated by pressure-driven myogenic response, the pathogenesis of focal changes remains debated. By AO, FANs and AVNs showed distinct anatomical features. At sites of FANs, the inner and outer limits of the arteriolar wall maintained their parallelism, and there was no evidence of parietal growth, suggesting that FANs were caused by focal vasoconstriction. In the microenvironment of AVNs, AO revealed a combination of loss of retinal transparency (Fig. 7.6) and presence of focal venous narrowings upstream and downstream of the arteriovenous crossing. The latter findings are in accordance with histology reports, which emphasized the role of the periarteriolar retina in the venous damage [9–11].

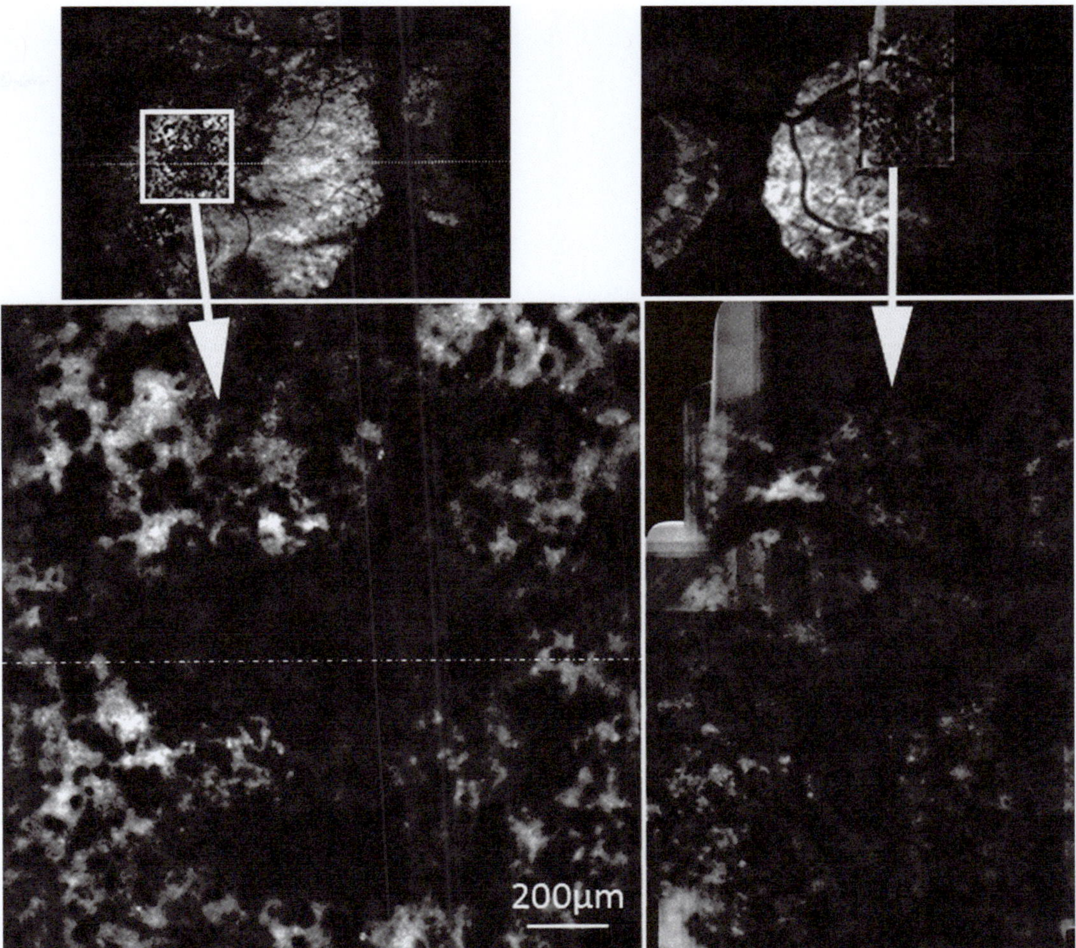

Fig. 7.4 GA case with foveal sparing. Note in the AO image the clear delineation of the area of preserved fovea

Diabetic retinopathy is also a leading cause of vision loss, especially in the working-age class. By AO imaging, microaneurysms and hemorrhages can be accurately diagnosed (Fig. 7.7). In some cases, parietal structures of microaneurysms could be observed.

7.4 Discussion

We show here that changes affecting the RPE or the structure of microvessels may be accurately documented using AO imaging. In GA cases, this allowed detection of very small spots of atrophy and follow-up of their progression but also the detection of RPE damage within as well as outside GA areas. It is indeed likely that the hyporeflective spots seen by AO correspond to melanin, given the known absorption-reflection profile of melanin [12]. Imaging of melanin redistribution is of interest because early AMD is associated with dysmorphic RPE and other cells containing melanosomes as part of presumed clearance activities [13–15]. Accurate characterization of the progression of atrophic lesions during GA is important for the estimation of its long-term prognosis and consequently for the evaluation of therapeutic results. It is likely that improved imaging of small GA lesions may allow evaluating the effect of treatment at earlier stages of the

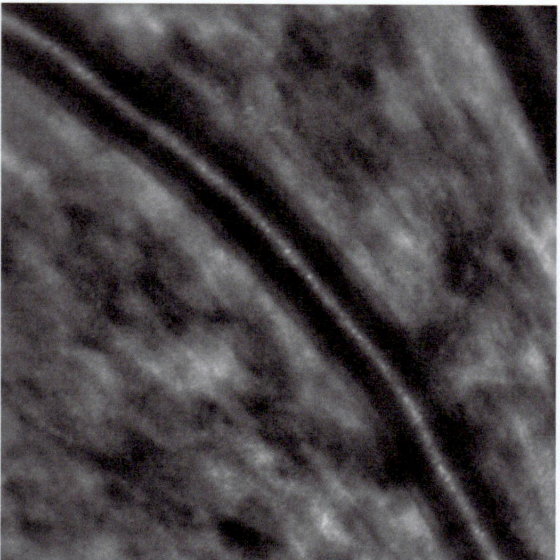

Fig. 7.5 AO imaging of a retinal artery showing the vessel wall

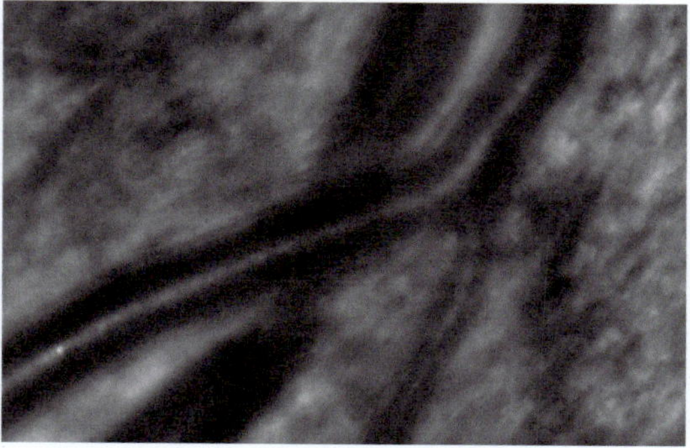

Fig. 7.6 AO imaging of arteriovenous nicking. Note that the arteriolar wall does not account for the blurring of the underlying vein

disease, where such treatment may be more susceptible to show efficacy. Additional studies are needed to clarify if isolated pigment deposits that can be seen in patients free of AMD are indicative of the risk of developing GA.

Vascular imaging offers also a new field of exploration for AO imaging, which is the only technique allowing a direct view of parietal structures. The light reflected back from the RPE probably contributes to parietal imaging [16]. Focal as well as diffuse changes can be observed. AO imaging of retinal arterioles also offers a unique

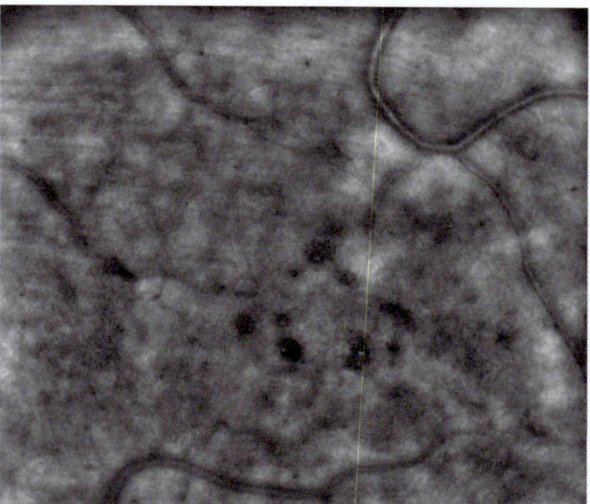

Fig. 7.7 AO imaging of diabetic microaneurysms

opportunity to explore age-, diabetes-, and hypertension-related microvascular changes in vivo in humans at a near-histology level. Phenotyping of retinal vessels by AO imaging may contribute to a better management and understanding of end-organ damage, especially in the brain given the functional and anatomical similarities of the retinal and cerebral circulations. Stratification of end-organ damage risk may be improved by biomarkers issued from AO imaging.

Up to now, the main application of AO fundus imaging has been photoreceptor detection and counting; this somewhat overshadowed the exploration of other retinal structures. With a simple procedure applicable in a routine setting, AO imaging can document microscopic features of common diseases such as GA, hypertensive retinopathy, and diabetic retinopathy and will possibly become a reference tool for their monitoring.

References

1. Liang J, Williams DR, Miller DT. Supernormal vision and high-resolution retinal imaging through adaptive optics. J Opt Soc Am A. 1997;14(11):2884–92.
2. Gocho K, Sarda V, Falah S, Sahel JA, Sennlaub F, Benchaboune M, et al. Adaptive optics imaging of geographic atrophy. Invest Ophthalmol Vis Sci. 2013; 54:3673–80.

3. Buus NH, Mathiassen ON, Fenger-Grøn M, Præstholm MN, Sihm I, Thybo NK, et al. Small artery structure during antihypertensive therapy is an independent predictor of cardiovascular events in essential hypertension. J Hypertens. 2013;31:791–7.
4. Wong TY, Klein R, Sharrett AR, Duncan BB, Couper DJ, Klein BE, et al. Atherosclerosis Risk in Communities Study. Retinal arteriolar diameter and risk for hypertension. Ann Intern Med. 2004;140:248–55.
5. Wong TY, Klein R, Nieto FJ, Klein BE, Sharrett AR, Meuer SM, et al. Retinal microvascular abnormalities and 10-year cardiovascular mortality: a population-based case–control study. Ophthalmology. 2003;110: 933–40.
6. Lindley RI, Wang JJ, Wong MC, Mitchell P, Liew G, Hand P, et al. Multi-Centre Retina and Stroke Study (MCRS) Collaborative Group. Retinal microvasculature in acute lacunar stroke: a cross-sectional study. Lancet Neurol. 2009;8:628–34.
7. Koch E, Rosenbaum D, Brolly A, Sahel JA, Chaumet-Riffaud P, Girerd X, Rossant F, Paques M. Morphometric analysis of small arteries in the human retina using adaptive optics imaging: relationship with blood pressure and focal vascular changes. J Hypertens. 2014;32:890–8.
8. Heagerty AM. Predicting hypertension complications from small artery structure. J Hypertens. 2007;25: 939–40.
9. Seitz R. The retinal vessels: comparative ophthalmoscopic and histologic studies on healthy and diseased eye. Translated by Frederick C. Blodi. Saint-Louis: CV Mosby; 1964.
10. Jefferies P, Clemett R, Day T. An anatomical study of retinal arteriovenous crossings and their role in the pathogenesis of retinal branch vein occlusions. Aust N Z J Ophthalmol. 1993;21:213–7.
11. Kimura T, Mizota A, Fujimoto N, Tsuyama Y. Light and electron microscopic studies on human retinal blood vessels of patients with sclerosis and hypertension. Int Ophthalmol. 2005;4:151–8.
12. Schmitz-Valckenberg S, Lara D, Nizari S, Normando EM, Guo L, Wegener AR, et al. Localisation and significance of in vivo near-infrared autofluorescent signal in retinal imaging. Br J Ophthalmol. 2011;95: 1134–9.
13. Cherepanoff S, McMenamin P, Gillies MC, Kettle E, Sarks SH. Bruch's membrane and choroidal macrophages in early and advanced age-related macular degeneration. Br J Ophthalmol. 2010;94:918–25.
14. Paques M, Simonutti M, Augustin S, Goupille O, El Mathari B, Sahel JA. In vivo observation of the locomotion of microglial cells in the retina. Glia. 2010;58: 1663–8.
15. Sarks SH. Ageing and degeneration in the macular region: a clinico-pathological study. Br J Ophthalmol. 1976;60:324–41.
16. Chui TY, Vannasdale DA, Burns SA. The use of forward scatter to improve retinal vascular imaging with an adaptive optics scanning laser ophthalmoscope. Biomed Opt Express. 2012;10:2537–49.

e-Learning by the Open-Access Journal *Atlas of Ophthalmology*

Georg Michelson and Moritz Michelson

8

Contents

G. Michelson, MD (⊠)
Verlag ONJOPH.COM, Erlangen, Germany

Department of Ophthalmology, Interdisciplinary
Center of Ophthalmic Preventive Medicine
and Imaging, Friedrich-Alexander University
Erlangen-Nürnberg, Schwabachanlage 6,
Erlangen 91054, Germany
e-mail: Georg.michelson@uk-erlangen.de

M. Michelson
Verlag ONJOPH.COM, Erlangen, Germany
e-mail: Moritz.michelson@t-online.de

8.1   Background

To prevent vision-threatening eye diseases in non-industrialized countries, a continuous medical education is necessary. Medical basic and advanced training in ophthalmology is strongly shaped by medical cases and pictures. Medical students and interns of ophthalmology in nonindustrialized countries often have inadequate access to illustrations of normal and rare diseases. Induced by consistently shortening time slices for complete renewal of medical knowledge, an increasing necessity for a continuous medical training evolves. In this context legal requirements with respect to medical training have been redefined in many countries [1–7]. Physicians are indebted by the Medical Association's professional code of conduct to improve their skills. Physicians, who are performing their profession, are obligated by the Medical Association's professional code of conduct to improve their skills to the extent necessary for the maintenance and development of essential specific skills they need for their profession. Physicians have to provide proof of their medical training to the medical association. Physicians, who document their voluntary further education, may apply for a certification of advanced training at the responsible medical association. In Germany the certification of advanced training enables physicians to record their regular qualified further education as a component of quality assurance (§ 5 of the German Medical Association's professional code of conduct) [8]. Additionally, the obligation

G. Michelson (ed.), *Teleophthalmology in Preventive Medicine*,
DOI 10.1007/978-3-662-44975-2_8, © Springer-Verlag Berlin Heidelberg 2015

of a professional to further training is determined in Book V of the German Social Welfare Code [9].

Currently, the health-care system underlies strong changes in the face of new communication channels because modern technologies of information and communication are integrated in many areas of the health-care system. The mode of further medical education changes with the use of the Internet and its associated multimedia-based possibilities. The application of new telecommunications may reshape presentations for continuing medical education or review articles about multimedia-based modules of advanced training. Recent research reported that Web 2.0 may be a useful mechanism for knowledge transfer [10].

Social media brings a new dimension to health care, offering a platform used by the public, patients, and health professionals to communicate about health issues with the possibility of potentially improving health outcomes.

8.2 Purpose and Main Outcome Measure

To quantity the worldwide acceptance of the social media platform of the open-access journal *Atlas of Ophthalmology* publishing ophthalmic case reports specified for the different access channels.

8.3 Methods

8.3.1 Technology

The technical fundamentals of the medical cases and pictures were in a SQL-based data bank containing dynamically generated websites. The search for pictures, submission, review, administration, and editing of picture contributions were effected by JAVA-supported online tools.

8.3.2 Access to the Database

The social media platform *Atlas of Ophthalmology* presented the cases within four different channels:

original website, Facebook, iPhone and iPad application, and Atlas 2.0 version.

The first and major access to cases and images was the website http://www.atlasophthalmology. com. Figure 8.1 depicts the screenshot of the start website. Under atlasophthalmology.com, ophthalmic cases reported were provided in English, German, Spanish, Russian, and Arabian language. The presentation of cases in the languages Japanese, Chinese, and Portuguese is in preparation.

8.3.3 Mode of Medical Case Presentation

In all four access channels, the case reports were presented by authors, diagnosis, comment, images, ICD code, and keywords. Each case was commented briefly and keywords were provided. More than 2,000 cases with about 9,200 pictures were accessible comprising the whole spectrum of ophthalmology. Navigation through the atlas was adapted to the well-known "arborization structure" of the Windows Explorer. For a better overview each picture was first displayed as a thumbnail (Fig. 8.2). Two different resolutions were provided, which were saved in JPEG format of 300 dpi for a quick overview and as a high-resolution image of 650 dpi. The high-resolution images were only available after registration. Each case and picture was provided with information about the author and institution. By means of an electronic watermark, the origin of the atlas pictures remained verifiable and detectable at any time.

8.3.4 Order of Cases

The cases were classified according to anatomical criteria: lids, conjunctiva, cornea, and so on. All cases were arranged strictly in the related folders according to a diagnosis key (Fig. 8.3). Additionally, in the Atlas 2.0 version, cases were presented by date of publishing (issue, according to the date of publication).

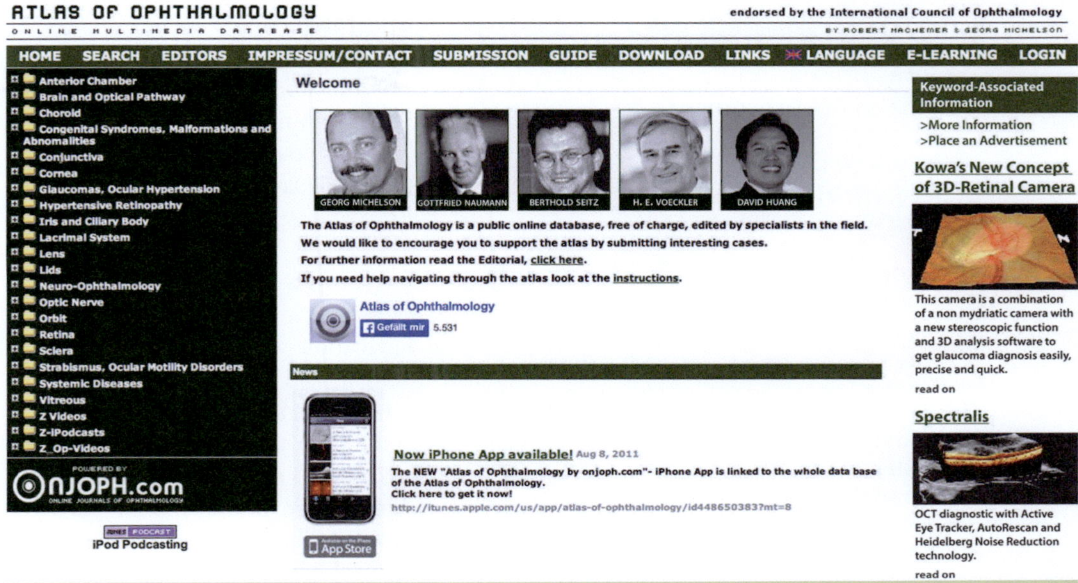

Fig. 8.1 Start page providing the task list SEARCH, EDITORIAL BOARD, CONTACT, SUBMISSION, HANDBOOK, DOWNLOAD, LINKS, LANGUAGE, e-LEARNING, and LOGIN, showing the portraits of the editorial board, the anatomical order of ophthalmic diseases, the direct link to the Facebook channel, the area of "keyword-associated information" as advertisement, and latest news (Reprinted with permission from Verlag ONJOPH.COM)

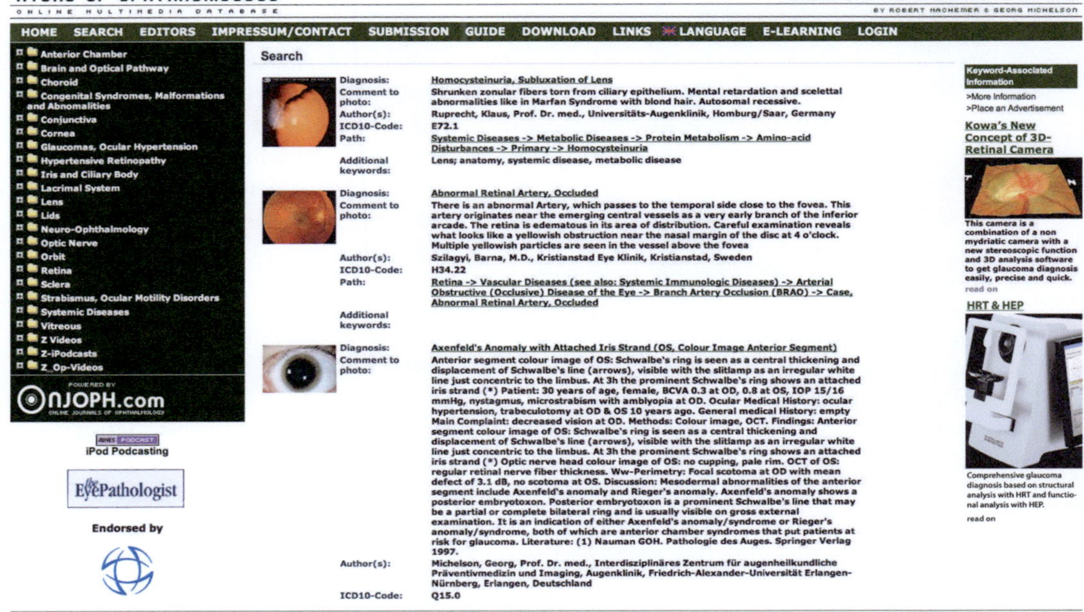

Fig. 8.2 Navigation through the atlas was adapted to the well-known "arborization structure" by Windows Explorer. For a better overview, each image was first displayed as a thumbnail (Reprinted with permission from Verlag ONJOPH.COM)

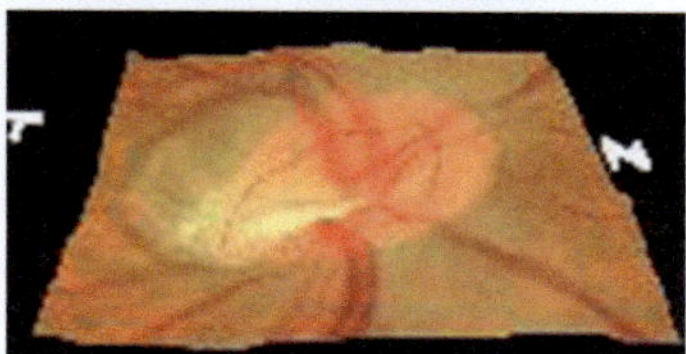

Fig. 8.3 Image depicts the placement of the advertisement with "keyword-associated information." The advertisement was presented by title, image, short text, and link (Reprinted with permission from Verlag ONJOPH.COM)

8.3.5 Navigation and Search Function

A fast query function and a complex search engine existed exhibiting several search modes. Cases and pictures could be searched by author, diagnosis, ICD code, and keywords.

8.3.6 Languages

Text and navigation was in Arabian, German, English, Russian, and Spanish, and, in part, in Portuguese, Japanese, and Chinese language. For each item of the atlas, the desired language could be selected. The total navigation, the diagnoses, and the comments were drafted multilingual. The atlas was presented completely in five languages, German, English, Spanish, Russian, and Arabian. Translation into the languages Portuguese, Chinese, and Japanese was partially completed. The translators were for English, H.E. Voelcker and Juliane Schlomberg; for Portuguese, Renato W. Damasceno; for German, Juliane Schlomberg; for Spanish, Raphael Cortez; for Chinese, Yanyan Koenig, Wu Liu, Qisheng You, and Liang Xu; for Russian, Alla Lisochkina; and for Arabic, Abdullah A. Laftal, Ahmad Wali, Abdullah Wali, Abdulwahed Mohammad Al-Amri, Osamah Al-Ghamdi, Mohammad Alhussain Alneamy, Ziyad Alhawali, Mohammed Alhefzi, Turki AL-Aziz, Muayyad Alhefdhi, Saqer Al-Deraan, Turki Dhafer Al-Shehri, and Mohammed Hammad ALMakady.

8.3.7 Submission

Only by the access channels http://www. atlasophthalmology.com and Atlas 2.0 version, the submission of cases was performed by documenting author(s), institution, email address, diagnosis, ICD-10 code, comment, and keywords. Online submission was organized as simple upload of pictures, authors, diagnosis, ICD code, and short comment. The entire process of peer review and publication was conducted online. Ophthalmologists of more than 156 countries submitted cases.

8.3.8 Review of Submitted Cases

Every case was reviewed by one of the editors before publication. Editors were G.O.H. Naumann [11], H.E. Völcker, D. Huang, B. Seitz, and G. Michelson. All cases and pictures submitted for publication underwent the online review process by the editors. Only accepted cases were published. The process of submission and review was effected online.

8.3.9 Certified Medical Education

A continuous medical education was implemented in the channel www.atlasophthalmology.com. The medical education tool was generated within an official cooperation with the "Bayerische Landesärztekammer." The e-learning system offered 21 modules. Every module contained medical cases of a distinct anatomical area of the eye (e.g., sclera, cornea, choroid). Per module three official CME points could be reached. To test the educational success, the user was asked to mark the correct diagnosis of ten clinical images, which were shown with five optional diagnoses. Only one of these five suggestions was the correct diagnosis. When more than 7 out of 10 questions were answered correctly, the users have reached 2 CME points. When all 10 questions were correctly answered, in total 3 CME points were released. After finishing the test, the certificate was sent to the user by email as a pdf document. The cost to perform one module was 4.99 €, payable through PayPal or by a voucher. The voucher contained a 12-digit number allowing the entrance to the e-learning system to complete one module.

8.3.10 Funding

Funding was predominantly by voluntary dedication. The funding of the open-access journal *Atlas of Ophthalmology* resulted from the voluntary work of editors, reviewers, authors, and coworkers and in part by support through advertisement by using the "keyword-associated information system."

8.3.11 Advertisement

In the access channel www.atlasophthalmology.com, industrial advertisement was presented as "keyword-associated information." The purpose of this service was to offer additional information to the selected medical case which was searched by the user. This information was displayed along with the search results. When a visitor searched images using distinct keywords, only an advertisement coupled with these keywords became visible for this user. The "keyword-associated information" appeared in the right column of the website. The advantage from this type of advertisement was that the information was only presented to the users interested in images which were coupled with the keywords of the advertisement. The "keyword-associated information" format included headline, small image, text, and a link to a website. Figure 8.3 depicts the placement of the "keyword-associated information."

8.3.12 Additional Access Channels

The *second access channel* of the social media platform was Facebook. Under www.facebook.com/AtlasOphthalmology, a selection of interesting cases was presented as *case of the week*, with only one image per case and exclusively in English language. Here the case was presented in a shortened version with only one image and a link to the original website atlasophthalmology.com presenting the complete case. Figure 8.4 showed a typical case presentation in Facebook. The *third access channel* to the medical cases was the iPhone and iPad application, presenting all published cases in English, German, Spanish, Russian, and Arabian language. These applications enabled a fast and mobile search of ocular diseases. The applications allowed a search for cases using diagnosis, ICD, or authors. The cases were presented by diagnosis, ICD code, comment, authors, and pictures given in middle or high resolution. Figures 8.5 and 8.6 depict the screenshots of the iPad and iPhone application, respectively. The applications could be downloaded from iTunes under the keyword "atlasophthalmology" – https://itunes.apple.com/us/app/atlas-of-ophthalmology/id448650383?mt=8.

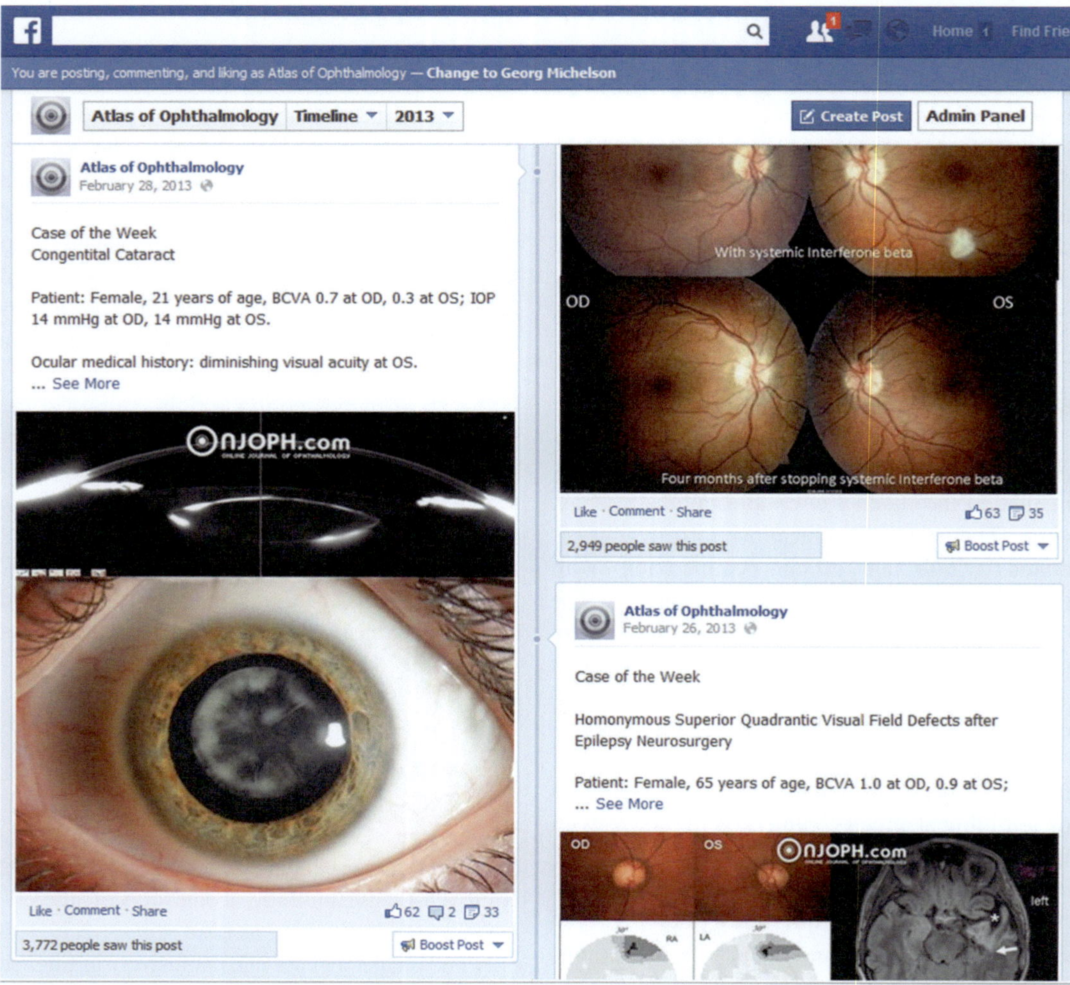

Fig. 8.4 The access channel Facebook presented the cases in a shortened version with a link to the complete case presentation under www.atlasophthalmology.com (Reprinted with permission from Verlag ONJOPH.COM)

The *fourth access channel* of the social media platform was the Atlas 2.0 version. Interactive and collaborative web applications offered new opportunities for reaching patients and other health-care consumers by facilitating information creation, sharing, and retrieval. Beginning in 2014 all medical cases were presented by the Web 2.0 technique, allowing a barrier-free access to the cases, independently of the browser or the used device such as a PC, tablet, or mobile phone. This technique enabled a full interactivity with the opportunity to discuss selected cases. The Atlas 2.0 version allowed to perform all process steps as submission, review, and publication according to MEDLINE and PubMed rules. Figure 8.7 represents screenshots of the *Atlas of Ophthalmology* 2.0.

8.3.13 Registration

To view images in the best resolution and to get permission to use images, a personal registration was needed. Only with an ID and password were these services available.

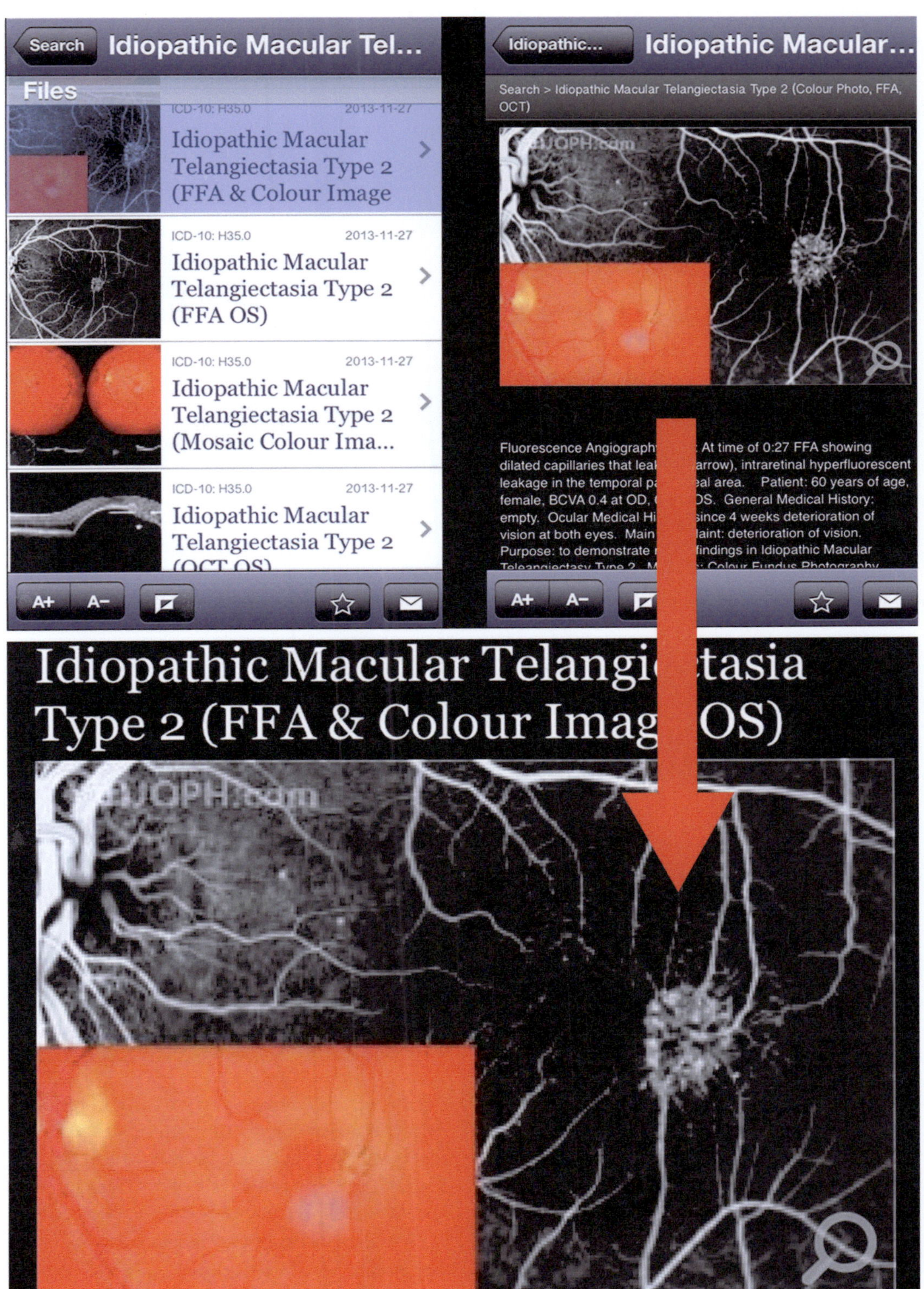

Fig. 8.5 iPad application: showing two screenshots of the iPad app "Atlas of Ophthalmology." The cases were presented by diagnosis, ICD code, image with comment, and authors. The app allowed to search for cases under diagnosis, ICD, and authors. All images were given in a middle or high resolution (Reprinted with permission from Verlag ONJOPH.COM)

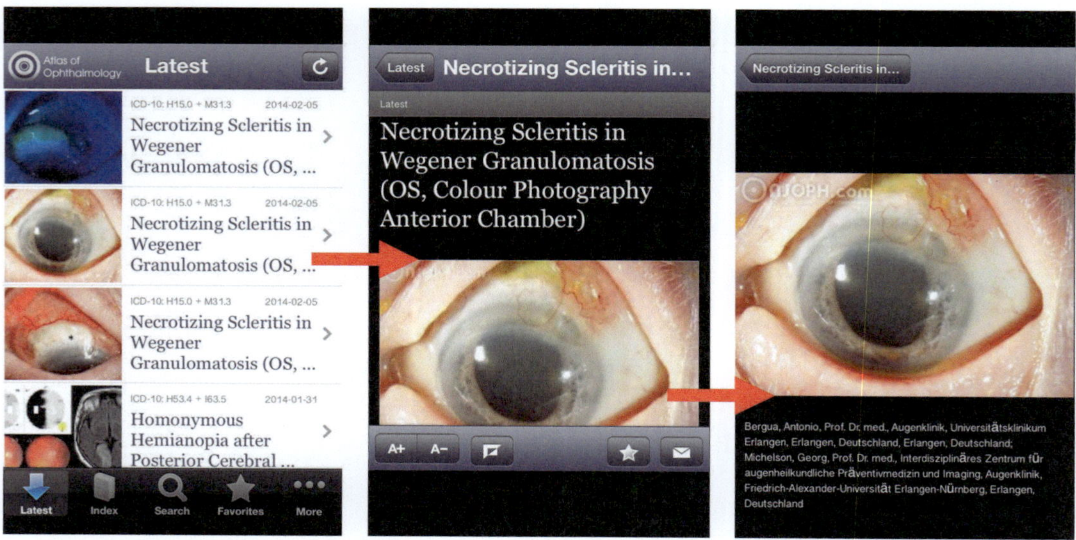

Fig. 8.6 Screenshots of the iPhone app. The cases were presented by diagnosis, ICD code, image with comment, and authors. By using the iPhone app, a fast and mobile search of ocular diseases can be performed (Reprinted with permission from Verlag ONJOPH.COM)

8.3.14 Statistics

Using the "Google statistics tool" and "Facebook page insights," analyses of the users were performed. Visitors data of 2013 from January to November were used.

8.4   Results

In 2013 (January 1st to November 30th), case reports and images were frequented in average by about 7.300 visitors per week, when summing up all three access channels of the social media platform. In order to use all the services, $N=14.000$ visitors were registered.

Visits by channel #1 (http://www. atlasophthalmology.com): In November 2013, $N=19.214$ people visited the site http://www. atlasophthalmology.com. $N=23.518$ visits and $N=169.369$ page views were documented. The site has had in average $N=5{,}595\pm315$ visitors per week from 166 countries coming predominantly from Germany (18 %), the USA (15 %), Japan (7 %), and Spanish-speaking countries (9.4 %). The distribution of used browsers was Chrome with 28 %, Internet Explorer with 26 %, Safari with 17 %, Firefox with 15 %, and Android Browser with 5 %. Table 8.1 specifies the countries where the most frequent users were coming from. The number of users using mobile techniques to get access to the main website was about 20 %. These visitors had an age lower than 35 years. Using the access http://www.atlasophthalmology.com, out of $N=23.518$ visits, $N=3.147$ visits were performed by iOS and $N=2.156$ visits by Android. Table 8.2 gives an overview of used mobile techniques having had access to http://www. atlasophthalmology.com.

Visits by channel #2 (www.facebook.com/ AtlasOphthalmology): In November 2013 the access channel Facebook has had a mean reach of $N=1{,}470\pm350$ subjects per week with $N=350\pm259$ post clicks per week, respectively. 91 % of the visitors of the Facebook channel have had an age lower than 35 years, and 48 % were female. The visitors (fans) were coming predominantly from the Arabian and Asian countries.

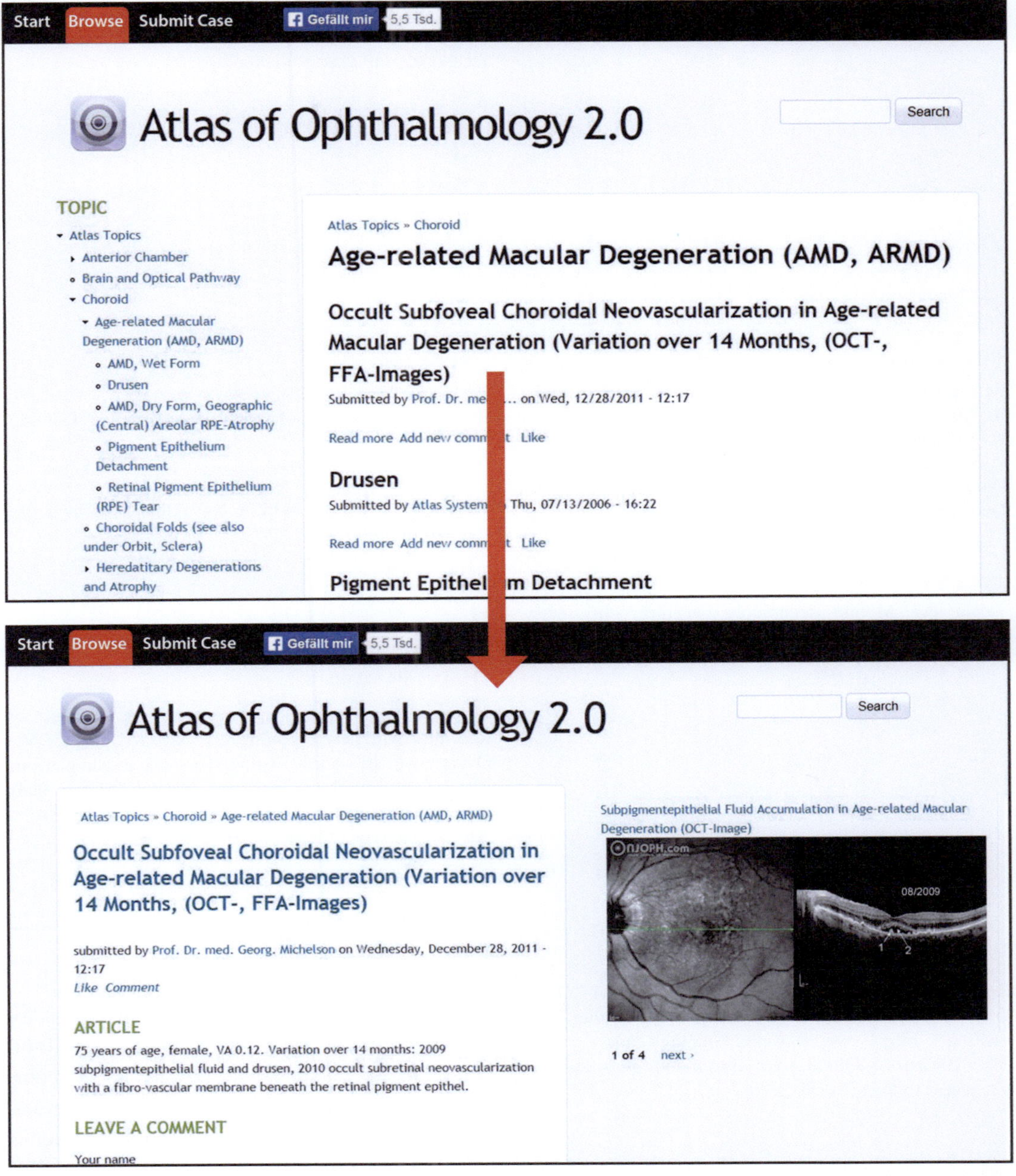

Fig. 8.7 *Atlas of Ophthalmology* 2.0: Using Web 2.0 technology navigation through the cases of Atlas 2.0 was possible by anatomical order or by issues according to the date of publication. Registered visitors could leave comments to distinct cases (Reprinted with permission from Verlag ONJOPH.COM)

The number of people who saw any activity from the page including posts, posts by other people, page-like ads, mentions, and check-ins was in average $N=393$ per day. Table 8.3 depicts the numbers of visitors of the Facebook channel by country of the month of November 2013.

*Visits by c*hannel #3 (iPhone and iPad application): In November 2013, in average $N=831$

Table 8.1 Visits in November 2013 using www.atlasophthalmology.com

	Country/territory	Visits	% Visits
1.	Germany	4,225	17.96
2.	United States	3,523	14.98
3.	Japan	1,831	7.79
4.	Russia	1,390	5.91
5.	Spain	1,389	5.91
6.	Mexico	856	3.64
7.	India	695	2.96
8.	United Kingdom	645	2.74
9.	Brazil	510	2.17
10.	Switzerland	498	2.12

Reprinted with permission from Verlag ONJOPH.COM
In November 2013, $N=19,214$ people visited the site www.atlasophthalmology.com with, in total, $N=23,518$ visits and $N=169,369$ page views. The main portion of visitors (more than 50 %) came from the countries Germany, the USA, Japan, Russia, and Spain

Table 8.2 Mobile techniques visiting http://www.atlasophthalmology.com in November 2013

	Operating system	Visits	% Visits
1.	iOS	3,147	56.37
2.	Android	2,156	38.62
3.	Windows Phone	111	1.99
4.	(Not set)	66	1.18
5.	BlackBerry	46	0.82
6.	Symbian OS	23	0.41
7.	Series 40	21	0.38
8.	Nokia	7	0.13
9.	Bada	4	0.07
10.	Samsung	1	0.02

Reprinted with permission from Verlag ONJOPH.COM
Overview of used mobile techniques in November 2013 visiting http://www.atlasophthalmology.com. About $N=5,200$ out of 23,000 users used mobile techniques to get access to the medical cases

unique visitors per week were documented, observing $N=4,577\pm135$ images per week using the iPhone and iPad application.

Summing up all access channels, $N=7,367$ unique visitors per week were documented. 65 % used the website www.atlasophthalmology, 24 % used Facebook, and 11 % used the iPhone application as access channel. Table 8.4 depicts the weekly visitors by type of access channel.

Table 8.3 Numbers of visitors of the Facebook channel of the month of November 2013 by country using www.facebook.com/atlasophthalmology

Country	Fans
Egypt	1,099
India	378
Pakistan	205
United States	192
Germany	187
Syria	181
Saudi Arabia	150
Libya	143
Russia	122
Iraq	115

Reprinted with permission from Verlag ONJOPH.COM

Table 8.4 Visits per week in November 2013 by access channel

Channel	Unique visitors per week	Percentage %
Website	4,793	65.0
Facebook	1,743	23.6
iPhone iPad app	831	11.4
Total	**7,367**	100

Reprinted with permission from Verlag ONJOPH.COM
Overview of all visitors visiting the social media platform *Atlas of Ophthalmology* by access channel. Here the number of weekly visitors of ophthalmic cases in November 2013 by the type of access

8.5 Discussion

There were limitations of the social media for health communication. The main recurring limitations of the social media are quality concerns and the lack of reliability of the health information. Authors of websites are often unidentifiable, or there can be numerous authors, or the line between producer and audience is blurred [12].

When using the described open-access journal *Atlas of Ophthalmology*, three overarching benefits can be identified: (1) The general public, patients, and health professionals have had the potential to increase the number of interactions and were provided with available, shared, and tailored information. (2) The medical content offered within our social media widened the access to those who may not easily access health information via traditional methods, such as younger people, ethnic minorities, and lower socioeconomic groups. (3) In addition we think that an important aspect of using our social media platform for ophthalmic health communication is that it provided valuable peer support for the general public and patients in respect to ocular diseases.

Ophthalmologic education in general is based largely on the visual evaluation of real medical cases and images. We intended to establish a worldwide multilingual open-access journal presenting ophthalmic case reports, which covers the whole field of ophthalmology. In November 2013 more than 2,000 cases were available by four different access channels, website http://www.atlasophthalmology.com, Facebook www.facebook.com/AtlasOphthalmology, iPhone and iPad application, and Atlas2.0 version. The major portion of users who visited the ophthalmic case collection by the website www.atlasophthalmology.com was 65 %. The access channel Facebook was used by a quarter of all visitors. The users of the Facebook channel predominantly came from Arabian and Asian countries.

In total and summing up all access channels, the average number of visits per week in November 2013 was about 7,300. The cases and images of the open-access journal *Atlas of Ophthalmology* were consulted in particular by faculty, residents, interns, medical students, and ancillary personnel for purposes of teaching and research. Due to the very comprehensive and well-assorted collection of cases and pictures, the atlas was used as a picture pool in the course of preparation of lectures. The use of pictures was free of charge for noncommercial purposes. Moreover, the pictures of the atlas were applied on different external websites as source of information. When images were needed for commercial purposes, the user had to pay for the download of the selected images. For noncommercial and commercial usage, a certificate for permission to use the images was necessary. Numerous benefits of using our social media platform for ophthalmic health communication were obvious for the general public, patients, and health professionals. A major benefit of the open-access journal *Atlas of Ophthalmology* for ophthalmic health communication was the accessibility and widening access of health information of ocular diseases to various population groups, regardless of age, education, race or ethnicity, and locality, compared to traditional communication methods.

Conclusion

The open-access journal *Atlas of Ophthalmology* publishing more than 2,000 cases with more than 9,000 images on the social media platform represented one of the most extensive and best commented collections of ophthalmologic images. In November 2013 the average number of visits per week was about 7,300, when summing up all three channels of access. About 14,000 registrations were documented. The case and picture database was available by four channels: by website http://www.atlasophthalmology.com, by Facebook www.facebook.com/AtlasOphthalmology, by an iPhone and iPad application, and by Atlas 2.0 version. Submission, review, and publication were performed completely by an online system. Google search listed the journal *Atlas of Ophthalmology* as number 1 with the comment "The Online Atlas of Ophthalmology is the biggest database with high-quality, peer-reviewed and commented pictures on the entire Internet."

References

1. De Silva DJ, Ramkissoon YD, Fielder AR. Skills acquired during training: a cause for concern? Br J Ophthalmol. 2007;91(9):1248–9.
2. International Task Force on Opthalmic Education of Medical Students, International Council of Opthalmology. Principles and guidelines of a curriculum for ophthalmic education of medical students. Klin Monatsbl Augenheilkd. 2006;223(Suppl 5):S1–19. http://www.icoph.org/med/preamble.html. Assessed 4 Feb 2009.
3. McDonnell PJ, Kirwan TJ, Brinton GS, Golnik KC, Melendez RF, Parke 2nd DW, Renucci A, Smith JH, Smith RE. Perceptions of recent ophthalmology residency graduates regarding preparation for practice. Ophthalmology. 2007;114(2):387–91.
4. Sherwin JC, Colville D. Ophthalmology education for Australian medical students. Clin Experiment Ophthalmol. 2008;36(5):491–2.

5. Ayaki M, Yaguchi S, Takagi Y, Matsuhashi M. Role of ophthalmology in the postgraduate medical training program. Nationwide survey and current problems. Jpn J Clin Ophthalmol. 2005;59(5):722–4.
6. Malik AS, Seng QB. Clinical experience of medical students in a developing country. Educ Health (Abingdon). 2003;16(2):163–75.
7. Gogate P, Deshpande M, Dharmadhikari S. Which is the best method to learn ophthalmology? Resident doctors' perspective of ophthalmology training. Indian J Ophthalmol. 2008;56(5):409–12.
8. German Medical Association. (Model) Regulations Continuing Education and Continuing Education Certificate (Art. 5). Available at: http://www.bundesaerztekammer.de/downloads/ADFBSatzungEn.pdf. Accessed 4 Feb 2009.
9. Deutsches Sozialgesetzbuch (SGB V – Gesetzliche Krankenversicherung, §§ 95d, 137) vom 20.12.1988. Available at: http://gesetze.bmas.de/Gesetze/gesetze.htm. Accessed 4 Feb 2009.
10. David I, Poissant L, Rochette A. Clinicians' expectations of web 2.0 as a mechanism for knowledge transfer of stroke best practices. J Med Internet Res. 2012;14(5):e121.
11. International Council of Ophthalmology. Ophthalmology continuing education programs and initiatives of the ICO. Available at: http://icoph.org/ed/icoce.html#atlas. Accessed 4 Feb 2009.
12. Moorhead SA, Hazlett DE, Harrison L, Carroll JK, Irwin A, Hoving C. A new dimension of health care: systematic review of the uses, benefits, and limitations of social media for health communication. J Med Internet Res. 2013;15(4):e85. doi:10.2196/jmir.1933.

Computer-Aided Diagnostics and Pattern Recognition: Automated Glaucoma Detection

9

Thomas Köhler, Rüdiger Bock, Joachim Hornegger, and Georg Michelson

Contents

T. Köhler, MSc (✉) • R. Bock
J. Hornegger, Dr.-Ing.
Pattern Recognition Lab, Department of
Computer Science, Friedrich-Alexander-Universität
Erlangen-Nürnberg, Erlangen, Bavaria, Germany

Erlangen Graduate School in Advanced Optical
Technologies (SAOT), Erlangen, Bavaria, Germany
e-mail: thomas.koehler@fau.de

G. Michelson, MD
Friedrich-Alexander-Universität Erlangen-Nürnberg,
Erlangen Graduate School in Advanced Optical
Technologies (SAOT), Erlangen, Bavaria, Germany

Department of Ophthalmology, Interdisciplinary
Center of Ophthalmic Preventive Medicine and
Imaging, Friedrich-Alexander-Universität Erlangen-
Nürnberg, Erlangen, Bavaria, Germany

9.1   Introduction

Glaucoma is a retinal disease influencing the *optic nerve head* (ONH) by damaging ganglion cells. Today, it is the second leading cause of blindness worldwide, affecting more than 60 million people in 2010. This number is estimated to increase to about 80 million in 2020 [1]. In the USA, more than 2.2 million people suffer from glaucoma, accounting for more than 9 % of all cases of blindness. In terms of economic impacts, this causes more than ten million physician visits and expenses of about US$1.5 billion per year [2].

The untreated glaucoma disease causes a successive degeneration of retinal nerve fibers particularly in the ONH region that leads to progressive narrowing of the visual field up to complete blindness. Proper treatment can stop the progress although already degenerated nerve fibers cannot be reactivated. Thus, the early detection and treatment of the disease are essential.

The initial diagnosis of glaucoma [3, 4] is extensive and consists of the assessment of:

1. Risk factors such as high intraocular pressure, race, age etc.
2. The front chamber angle
3. The morphology of the ONH (Sect. 9.4.1)
4. Possible defects of the visual field

Furthermore, a longitudinal assessment of the ONH is performed to confirm the initial diagnosis. Despite the steady rise of diseases over the past years, glaucoma is often undiagnosed until the unrecoverable structural damage of retinal nerve

G. Michelson (ed.), *Teleophthalmology in Preventive Medicine*,
DOI 10.1007/978-3-662-44975-2_9, © Springer-Verlag Berlin Heidelberg 2015

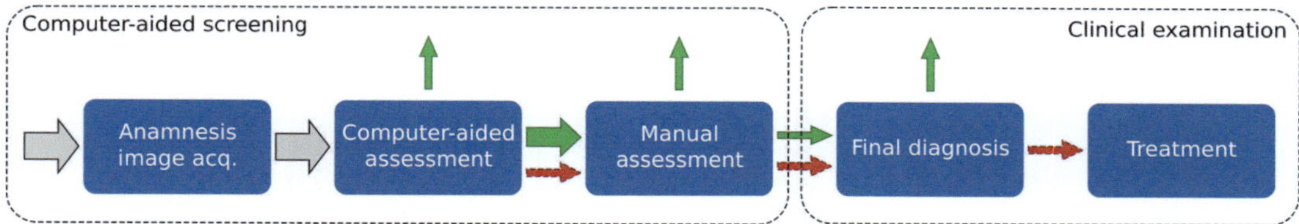

Fig. 9.1 Computer-aided screening consists of subsequent building blocks: Initially, the anamnesis and image data of the entire screening collective is analyzed to preselect unsuspicious cases. The remaining set has to be manually assessed for further exclusion of unremarkable subjects. Only a small proportion of the initial set will be forwarded to clinical assessment to gain a final diagnosis and follow-up treatment if necessary

fibers gets evident by the significant narrowing of the visual field. Several studies showed that screening programs for glaucoma [5] can reduce this high number of unreported cases. The main goal of these screening applications is the detection of suspicious cases from a large population and their successful routing to more extensive clinical examination for a final diagnosis. Common screening populations are characterized by a high amount of normals which have to be assessed manually by the involved reading center (Fig. 9.1 step (3)).

Computer-aided diagnostics (CAD) supports an ophthalmologist in the preparation of a medical diagnosis based on automatic data-mining methods. In particular, CAD is applicable in screening setups in order to reduce the number of normals for manual judgment, which helps to increase the efficiency of the reading centers (Fig. 9.1 step (2)). This is done by an upstream analysis of the personal data, e.g. images or anamnesis data, utilizing pattern recognition techniques that automatically perform a preselection of suspicious cases. Here, a computer-aided assessment augments the manual assessment provided by the reading center. As depicted in Fig. 9.1, this approach is considered as *computer-aided screening* (CAS). The proposed strategy can also be realized in a telemedical setup where image acquisition and examination are done spatially and temporally separated.

Scope

This contribution provides an overview on the recent advances in the development of pattern recognition techniques for automatic glaucoma detection. We will focus on fully automatic techniques applicable within a screening environment utilizing pure structural retinal fundus data published in 2008 or later.

Outline

The remainder of this chapter is organized as follows: After the introduction of common imaging modalities to document ONH morphology, we provide an excursus on pattern recognition. As major part of this work, two methodologies are presented that arise from current automatic glaucoma detection literature on structural retinal image data: (i) structure-driven and (ii) data-driven techniques. Finally, the methods are compared and evaluated toward the application in CAS.

9.2 Imaging Modalities

One main part in diagnosing glaucoma is the assessment of the ONH morphology. Besides the slit lamp that allows a live examination of the eye background, several digital imaging modalities got established. These devices allow the documentation of the ONH's structure by acquiring 2-dimensional (2-D) or 3-dimensional (3-D) image data as shown in Fig. 9.2.

Fundus imaging is one of the most commonly used technologies in ophthalmology to obtain high-resolution color photographs of the human retina [7, 8]. The fast image acquisition and relatively low costs of a digital fundus camera make this modality attractive to document the retina during screening. The acquired images can be analyzed to detect pathological degenerations caused, e.g., by glaucoma [9].

Confocal laser ophthalmoscope commercially available as *Heidelberg retina tomograph* (HRT) [10] acquires topographic and gray-scaled reflectance images of the ONH. In particular, the topographic images capturing the ONH's shape allow the extraction of parameters to discriminate between normals and glaucomatous subjects [11].

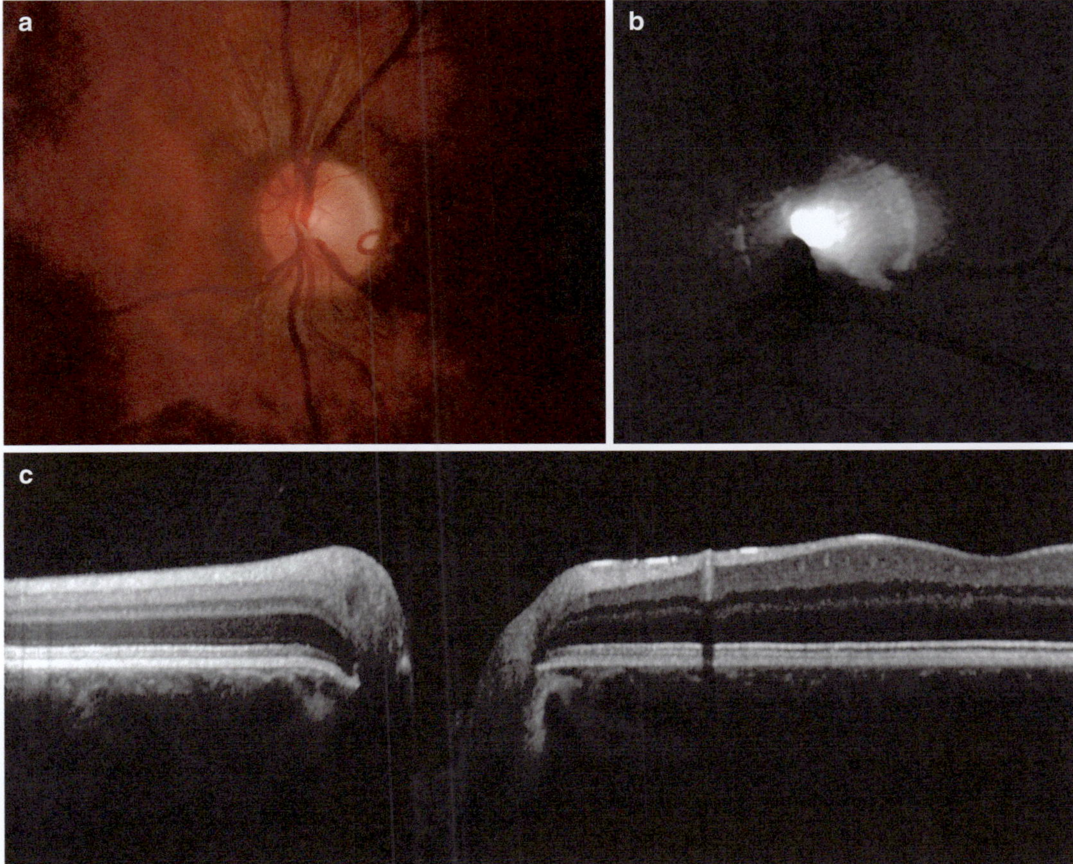

Fig. 9.2 Sample images capturing the optic nerve head (ONH) region: (**a**) high-resolution color fundus image, (**b**) topographic image acquired with Heidelberg retina tomograph (HRT), and (**c**) OCT line scan intersecting the ONH and depicting the different retinal layers including the retinal nerve fiber layer as the top one (Reprinted from [6] with permission from Elsevier)

Optical coherence tomography (OCT) [12] as the optical pendant to ultrasound enables the acquisition of depth profiles and even entire 3-D volumes of the retina. As the image data also records the *retinal nerve fiber layer* (RNFL), OCT data allows a detailed judgment of the retinal constitution and a reliable diagnosis of glaucoma. In addition, OCT data can be utilized for CAD applications as it was demonstrated by Huang and Chen [13] and Burgansky et al. [14]. As an alternative device for measuring the RNFL thickness, also scanning laser polarimetry (SLP) can be utilized.

From this retinal image data, pattern recognition techniques can extract glaucoma-related markers utilized during the computer-aided assessment within a screening scenario as shown in Fig. 9.1.

9.3 Excursus: Pattern Recognition Pipeline

The goal of pattern recognition is to analyze and classify patterns such as images or speech. For this purpose, pattern recognition systems are divided into multiple processing stages that are organized as a pipeline with similar underlying structure for different real-world problems [15]. In terms of glaucoma detection based on retinal image data, this pipeline is outlined in Fig. 9.3. Please also refer to Fig. 9.1 as the pattern recognition pipeline can be embedded within the automated glaucoma assessment step.

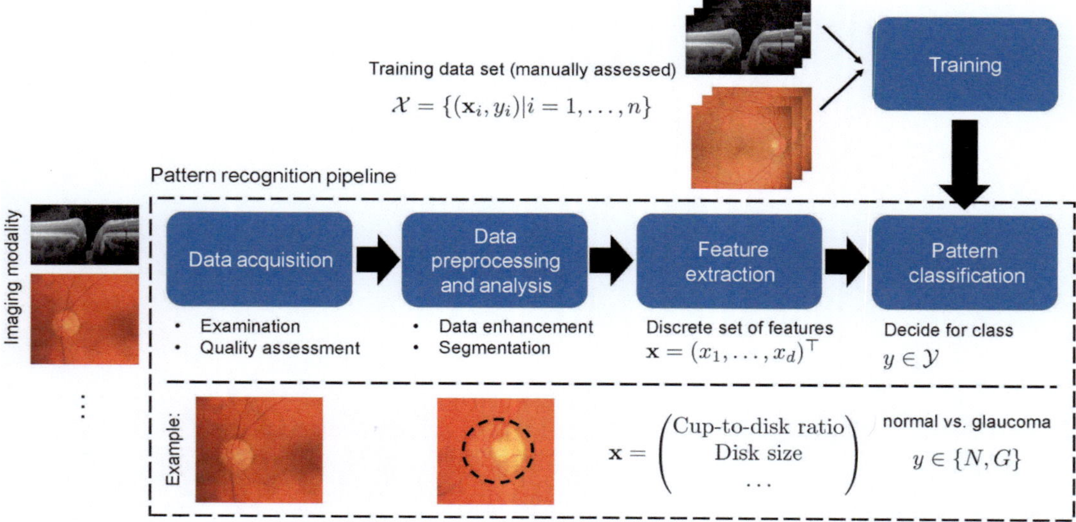

Fig. 9.3 Pattern recognition pipeline applied to automated glaucoma detection: Retinal image data is (i) acquired with an eye imaging modality such as fundus imaging or optical coherence tomography (OCT), (ii) preprocessed and analyzed as preparation for pattern recognition techniques, (iii) used to extract relevant features to detect traces of glaucoma, and (iv) used in a classification stage trained with manually classified image data. A common example workflow is visualized for glaucoma detection based on fundus photographs

Data Acquisition

In an initial data acquisition stage, sensor data such as images or speech is captured. Analog sensor data is commonly converted into a *discrete* mathematical representation for further processing by means of pattern recognition methods.

Example: For image-based glaucoma detection, the human eye is captured with an imaging modality. In a common clinical workflow, digital fundus cameras are employed to analyze the optic nerve for traces of glaucoma. As glaucoma detection relies on the quality of the acquired image, data acquisition also involves quality assessment for image data. In case of fundus imaging, several automatic and objective quality indices have been proposed to recognize images not usable for further processing [16–18].

Data Preprocessing and Analysis

Pattern recognition techniques require an appropriate preparation of the acquired data. Therefore, preprocessing steps are required to correct invalid or erroneous measurements present in the raw data. Different parts of the acquired signal that are relevant for a specific pattern recognition problem are extracted and analyzed. Then, these parts are used to measure certain parameters and to classify patterns in the underlying sensor data.

Example: Retinal image analysis [19] provides methods to process and analyze retinal image data in order to measure clinical parameters of the eye. In terms of fundus imaging, preprocessing for image enhancement includes illumination correction [20] to adjust uneven contrast and denoising techniques [21] to enhance the quality of noisy data. Preprocessing is also beneficial to remove features not related to glaucoma and to make the measurement of disease-specific parameters more reliable [22]. Common analysis steps include a segmentation of the ONH for glaucoma assessment [23–25].

Feature Extraction

Feature extraction reduces the complexity of the prepared data by modeling it with a finite set of features organized as a *feature vector* $\mathbf{x} \in \mathbf{R}^d$. Each single feature x_i is a mathematical description of a certain parameter or measurement. Features can be either continuous, e.g., geometric measurements such as lengths or diameters of anatomical structures, or discrete, e.g., the sex of a human subject. Additionally, dimensionality reduction may be used in an optional step to reduce the complexity of raw features $\mathbf{x}$ to obtain a compressed feature vector $\mathbf{x}' \in {}^{d'}$ where $d' < d$. Feature selection techniques learn the most meaningful features $\mathbf{x}'$ in an automatic manner based on example data. Opposed to this approach, *principal component analysis* (PCA) is a common tool to perform dimensionality reduction in an unsupervised procedure.

Example: Features that can be extracted from fundus images are geometric parameters of the ONH segmented in the previous stage of the pipeline. This includes the well-known *cup-to-disk ratio* (CDR) denoted as x_1 or the size of the optic disk denoted as x_2. The associated feature vector is given by $\mathbf{x} = (x_1, x_2)^\mathsf{T}$.

Pattern Classification

Sensor data represented by a feature vector $\mathbf{x}$ is characterized by a *class label* $y \in \mathcal{Y}$ where $\mathcal{Y} = \{y_1, \ldots, y_k\}$ denotes a discrete set of k classes. However, the true class label is unknown and must be determined from the features. A *classifier* predicts a class label y^* from the features $\mathbf{x}$ in an automatic manner. Therefore, the classifier is derived from a *training set* $\mathcal{X} = \{(\mathbf{x}_i, y_i) \mid i = 1, \ldots, n\}$ to learn the relationship between the features $\mathbf{x}_i$ and the associated class y_i. The set $\mathcal{X}$ is composed from n training patterns $\mathbf{x}_1, \ldots, \mathbf{x}_n$, where the true class label y_i for each $\mathbf{x}_i$ is known and is used as gold standard. State-of-the-art classifiers commonly used in practical applications are support vector machines (SVM), random forests, artificial neural networks (ANN), or boosting methods such as AdaBoost [15].

Example: In glaucoma detection, we are interested in the state of glaucoma, and the aim is to solve a two-class problem with $y \in \{N, G\}$ whereas $y = N$ for a normal subject and $y = G$ for a subject suffering from glaucoma, respectively. Nayak et al. [9] proposed an ANN to discriminate between healthy normals and glaucomatous eyes based on features gained from fundus images. Therefore, the ANN is trained with patterns obtained from manually labeled fundus images provided by an ophthalmologist.

9.4 Glaucoma Detection by Means of Imaging

One trend in ophthalmology is the quantitative survey of the retinal fundus based on image data acquired in a noninvasive and in vivo way. These techniques utilize characteristics of the ONH as parameter and can be embedded within glaucoma screening programs [26]. As already depicted in Sect. 9.1, they can be automatically employed within a computer-aided assessment step to detect traces of glaucoma based on image data and to provide an initial exclusion of most likely normal cases.

Two major types of methodologies can be distinguished:

Structure-driven techniques commonly automate the extraction of established structural parameters of the ONH, e.g., the diameters of the optic disk and cup. These parameters are already known in the medical community and also statistically verified but are often determined manually.

Data-driven techniques utilize data-mining methods applied on the *entire* image to obtain discriminative markers for glaucoma detection. In contrast to structure-driven techniques, no direct relation between the ONH structure and the marker can be further obtained.

9.4.1 Structure-Driven Glaucoma Detection

In structure-driven glaucoma detection, disease-specific indicators of clinical significance are measured quantitatively. In general, glaucoma is characterized by a continuous, irreversible loss of ganglion cells [3]. This loss is the root cause for a set of structural ONH changes which can be captured by fundus imaging modalities as introduced in Sect. 9.2: (i) Thinning of the neuroretinal rim and (ii) a simultaneous extension of ONH cupping can be measured in fundus photographies and HRT images [27] as shown in Fig. 9.4 for an example fundus image [8]. (iii) The thinning of the retinal nerve fiber layer can be quantified, e.g., by OCT devices, and correlates with visual field defects due to glaucoma [28].

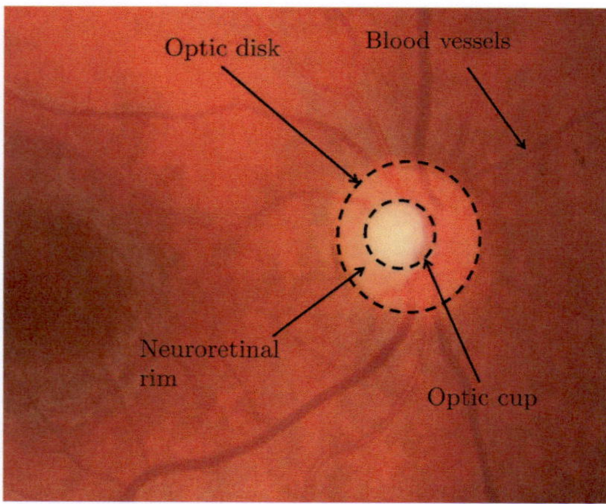

Fig. 9.4 Fundus image showing the optic nerve head (ONH): The optic cup is visible as bright spot inside the optic disk enclosed by the neuroretinal rim (Image data is taken from the high-resolution fundus (HRF) database

9.4.1.1 2-D Optic Nerve Head Analysis

A medically established feature accepted for glaucoma diagnosis is the *cup-to-disk ratio* (CDR) defined as:

$$CDR = \frac{d_{cup}}{d_{disk}} \qquad (9.1)$$

where d_{cup} and d_{disk} denote the vertical cup and disk diameter, respectively. With a thinned neuroretinal rim and an enlarged cup in case of glaucomatous eyes, a larger CDR indicates an increased risk of glaucoma.

Originally, the CDR was manually determined. An automated calculation is possible when utilizing recent image segmentation algorithms. A supervised procedure employs pixel classification to discriminate between disk, cup, and remaining background, e.g., based on superpixels [25]. Contrary, region-based methods rely on active contour models for disk segmentation and vessel-bend detection [23]. In case of stereo fundus imaging, the depth map obtained from a stereo image pair can be utilized to increase the reliability of the cup segmentation [29]. Once disk and cup are segmented, d_{cup} and d_{disk} are measured to determine the CDR according to Eq. (9.1).

The CDR may also be combined with further structural features such as the blood vessel areas

in *inferior, superior, nasal, and temporal* (ISNT) quadrants or the distance between optic disk center and ONH as proposed by Nayak et al. [9]. The optic disk size should also be included to glaucoma classification as it highly correlates with CDR [30].

9.4.1.2 Topographic Optic Nerve Head Analysis

One inherent limitation of the CDR is that it ignores the underlying surface of the ONH as it is a 2-D feature only. HRT imaging enables the topographic analysis of the optic nerve which has been also investigated for glaucoma detection [11, 31].

In the approach of Swindale et al. [11], a surface model $z:\ ^2 \rightarrow\ $ estimated from ONH images defines the depth z as a function of the position (u, v) on the ONH. This model consists of two parts modeling the surface: (i) the parabolic retinal fundus and (ii) the ONH cup, which is parameterized by ten features. These encode meaningful structural features such as center, radius, slope, or depth of the optic cup as well as secondary parameters such as cup gradient measures derived from the model. They differ for healthy and glaucomatous subjects and are utilized for glaucoma detection. The resulting *glaucoma probability score* (GPS) is obtained by a Bayes classifier which allows to introduce an adapted *loss functions* [15] in order to penalize a misclassification of a glaucoma patient as a healthy one, usually referred to as false negative. This is useful in a screening scenario where unrecognized cases should be avoided.

Twa et al. [32] modeled the ONH depth profile utilizing pseudo-Zernike radial polynomials. The parameters are then used as features within a decision tree classification. This method can be considered as a generalization of Swindale et al. [11] as a generic parametric function is used in comparison to a cup-specific parametric model.

9.4.1.3 Volumetric Retinal Nerve Fiber Layer Analysis

In addition to 2-D and topographic modalities, OCT imaging enables an in-depth analysis of the retinal layers. To enable a reliable determination of the RNFL, modality-specific image artifacts such as speckle noise [33–35] and motion artifacts [36] need to be compensated beforehand. Afterward, an automatic analysis of the RNFL by image processing and classification methods is promising for glaucoma detection [13, 14].

A threshold-based classification schema considering the single average RNFL thickness is proposed by Pachiyappan et al. [37]. The RNFL is automatically segmented by active contours.

The amount of input features is extended by Bizios et al. [38] who added new parameters to the conventional structural measurements that capture percentile thickness values of different retinal quadrants around the ONH. For classification, (i) an SVM and (ii) neural network classifiers were applied and compared.

An automatic framework for glaucoma detection that also extends the feature space has been proposed by Mayer et al. [39]. Based on an automatic segmentation of the RNFL in *circular B-scans* centered at the ONH [40], the following features are extracted from the RNFL thickness profile and used as classifier input: (i) statistical features including minimum, maximum, and mean values of the profile and (ii) the entire thickness profile compressed by a PCA model. The yielded feature vector **x** only represents the appearance of the RNFL without including any anamnesis data and is utilized by an SVM classifier.

Overall, the structure-driven methods for glaucoma detection mainly rely on a small set of highly discriminative and medically motivated features.

9.4.2 Data-Driven Glaucoma Detection

In data-driven approaches, the *entire* image data is exploited by general-purpose features such as spectral or texture features that are established in signal and image processing. These features are neither directly related to glaucoma nor of clinical meaningfulness but represent an abstract mathematical description of the retina. Novel techniques employing this concept for glaucoma detection are described in the following sections.

9.4.2.1 Higher-Order Spectra (HOS) and Texture Analysis

The glaucoma detection method introduced by Acharya et al. [41] exploits *higher-order spectra* (HOS) features that are combined with texture features.

The proposed HOS features exploit phase and amplitude information of fundus images. Spectral descriptors are obtained from this information and are used as features for glaucoma classification.

The variation of pixel values in an image encodes its texture. For the extraction of texture features, two quantities are analyzed:

(i) The *gray-level co-occurrence matrix* encodes the number of combinations for different pixel values in an image. Additionally, a difference matrix encodes probabilities that a certain gray-level differences between two pixels occur. This is derived from the co-occurrence matrix.

(ii) The *run-length matrix* $P_\theta(i, j)$ encodes how often a pixel value i successively appears j time for a certain direction given by angle θ. From these quantities, texture descriptors are derived as features. For a mathematical definition of the complete feature set, the interested reader is referred to [41].

HOS and texture features are combined as a joint feature set to discriminate healthy and glaucoma subjects. Therefore, SVM, random forests, and naive Bayes classifiers have been investigated showing competitive performance in terms of sensitivity and specificity.

9.4.2.2 Wavelet-Based Features

Dua et al. [42] proposed to use the *discrete wavelet transform* (DWT) as a feature extractor in glaucoma detection from fundus images showing the ONH.

The DWT decomposes the input signal, i.e., the fundus image, into spatial and frequency domains at different scalings and is well established in signal and image processing. To identify the most discriminative descriptors for glaucoma detection, this extensive set of features is then reduced by feature ranking and selection. Similar to [41], several classifiers such as random forest, SVM, and naive Bayes have been investigated.

9.4.2.3 Eigenimages and Glaucoma Risk Index (GRI)

The concept of appearance-based pattern recognition for glaucoma detection on fundus images was introduced by Bock et al. [6] and is inspired by the *Eigenimages* originally proposed for face recognition [43].

First, input images are preprocessed using ONH centering, illumination correction, and blood vessel inpainting to remove image characteristics not related to glaucoma. Then, three different feature types are extracted from the images: (i) the raw image intensities, (ii) the Fourier coefficients, and (iii) the B-spline coefficients. Each of these feature sets is separately compressed by an unsupervised PCA to condense the major image variations into a compact format. Finally, an SVM classifier hierarchy is employed. In the first stage, each feature vector per feature type is classified by one probabilistic SVM yielding three distinct glaucoma probabilities. In the second stage, these three probabilities are then merged to an intermediate feature vector and used as input for an additional probabilistic SVM to obtain a final probabilistic *glaucoma risk index* (GRI). The processing pipeline for the GRI computation is outlined in Fig. 9.5.

9.4.2.4 Independent Component Analysis

A further appearance-based method for glaucoma detection has been proposed by Fink et al. [44]. This method utilizes the *independent component analysis* (ICA) [45] on images captured with a confocal laser ophthalmoscope (Heidelberg retina tomograph (HRT)). In contrast to PCA, ICA decomposes the signal into statistically independent factors. The entire HRT image is treated as a feature vector and used to derive its ICA decomposition coefficients. The final classification is then achieved by applying a K-nearest neighbor classifier utilizing these coefficients as a feature.

9.5 Summary

This section summarizes the performance of the described structural and data-driven approaches. Subsequently, both paradigms are discussed and compared.

9.5.1 Performance Comparison

For quantitative evaluation, the following measurements are considered: (i) the accuracy to assess the percentage of correctly classified images, (ii) the sensitivity and specificity to quantify the trade-off between a sensitive glaucoma detection and an unreasonable high false-positive rate, and (iii) the area under the *receiver operating characteristic curve* (AUC) to evaluate for the overall performance. While the AUC measurement is independent from a binary cut-off threshold during classification, the remaining measurements might be adjusted by selecting a different threshold, e.g., optimized for a screening scenario. Table 9.1 summarizes quantitative results as reported in the cited original publications. The numbers are not necessarily gained from the same sample set and may have different distributions of

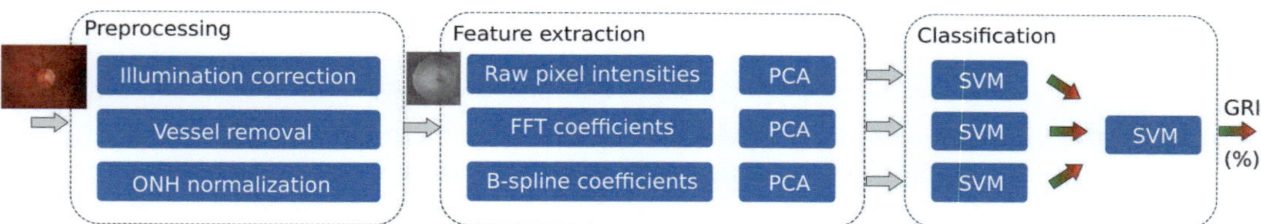

Fig. 9.5 Glaucoma risk index (*GRI*): The processing pipeline performs three major steps: (i) preprocessing to eliminate disease independent variations, (ii) data-driven feature extraction based on different feature types and principal component analysis (*PCA*), and (iii) two-stage probabilistic classification using support vector machine (*SVM*) to achieve the final risk index

Table 9.1 Summary of cited references for data-driven (*D*) and structure-driven (*S*) approaches. Imaging modalities utilized for glaucoma detection are fundus imaging (*FI*), the Heidelberg retina tomograph (*HRT*) for topographic analysis, and optical coherence tomography (*OCT*) for volumetric analysis. A measure is omitted (−) if it is not reported in the original publication

Method	S/D	Modality	Images	Sens. (%)	Spec. (%)	Acc. (%)	AUC (%)
Fundus images (2-D)							
Cheng et al. [25]	S	FI	2,326	−	−	−	82
Superpixels, cup-to-disk ratio (CDR)							
Nayak et al. [9]	S	FI	61	100	80	90	−
CDR, ISNT rule (inferior-superior-nasal-temporal)							
Acharya et al. [41]	D	FI	60	−	−	92	−
Higher-order spectra (HOS), texture							
Dua et al. [42]	D	FI	60	−	−	93	−
Wavelet							
Bock et al. [6]	D	FI	575	73	85	80	88
Eigenimages, principal component analysis (PCA)							
Topographic analysis							
Swindale et al. [11]	S	HRT	200	88	89	89	−
Glaucoma probability score (GPS)							
Twa et al. [32]	S	HRT	275	69	88	80	88
Zernike polynomial							
Fink et al. [44]	D	HRT	120	−	−	91	−
Independent component analysis (ICA)							
Volumetric analysis							
Bizios et al. [38]	S	OCT	152	−	−	−	98
Retinal nerve fiber layer (RNFL) measurements							
Mayer et al. [39, 40]	S/D	OCT	204	90	90	−	94
(RNFL, PCA)							

glaucoma disease, age, sex, or race. If multiple classifiers were evaluated on the same feature set, we report the best performance achieved.

The results indicate that image-based glaucoma detection achieves a notable accuracy and an AUC of at least 80 %, respectively. Considering fundus photography and HRT imaging, both structural and data-driven methods can achieve an accuracy of around 90 %. However, volumetric analysis based on OCT data is characterized by an outstanding AUC of up to 98 %. Thus, neither structural nor data-driven methodology is outperforming the other one, while the volumetric, structure-driven techniques seem to be most discriminative.

9.5.2 Structure-Driven vs. Data-Driven Approach

The presented paradigms achieve a comparable glaucoma detection performance within the same imaging modality although they both rely on contrary basic assumptions.

Structure-driven methods depend on a small, but highly discriminative, set of features, neglecting the bigger part of the image data. In general, these are either computed by fitting a parametric model to the image data or segmenting retinal structures. The obtained indicators were manually selected and proved by clinical studies and/or trials. In mass screening, an automated and reliable analysis, e.g., of the CDR, relies on an accurate segmentation of cup and disk. However, since boundaries of these structures are not well defined and highly variable, such an automatism is difficult to achieve in practice.

In data-driven approaches, no manual preselection of the image content is performed, but the entire image data is utilized. The desired compact set of discriminative features required for a reasonable classification is then obtained by a subsequent automatic feature selection and compression. Thus, the data-driven techniques might extract novel features that are not yet captured by structure-driven approaches. A further medical analysis of these data-driven features is promising as it might provide new insights to glaucoma disease and its variations.

Conclusion

This chapter presents novel trends for glaucoma detection by means of pattern recognition. These techniques employ noninvasive and in vivo imaging of the human retina and can be embedded to computer-aided screening. In the course of this chapter, methods based on fundus photography, topographic HRT imaging, and volumetric analysis using OCT are reviewed. The two major methodologies, i.e., (i) structure- and (ii) data-driven techniques, utilize complementary image information and showed a comparable performance.

Even when first experimental evaluations showed promising results, there are several ways to extend these techniques and to gain new insight to glaucoma disease and its characteristics. Since all presented methods employ a single imaging modality, multimodal techniques are an interesting extension. Therefore, complementary information, e.g., 2-D photometric data obtained from fundus photography augmented by volumetric data acquired by OCT, can be used to extract a multimodal feature set. In addition, features obtained by structural and data-driven methods can be combined to a hybrid classification approach. This might improve automatic glaucoma detection in order to reduce the amount of manually assessed screening patients and may help to reduce the costs of glaucoma screening programs.

Acknowledgment The authors gratefully acknowledge funding of the Erlangen Graduate School in Advanced Optical Technologies (SAOT) by the German National Science Foundation (DFG) in the framework of the excellence initiative.

References

1. Quigley HA, Broman AT. The number of people with glaucoma worldwide in 2010 and 2020. Br J Ophthalmol. 2006;90(3):262–7.
2. Glaucoma Research Foundation. Glaucoma facts and stats. 2013. Available from: http://www.glaucoma.org.
3. European Glaucoma Society, editor. Terminology and guidelines for glaucoma. 2nd ed. Savona: Editrice Dogma; 2003.

4. Bonomi L, Marchini G, Marraffa M, Bernardi P, De Franco I, Perfetti S, et al. Prevalence of glaucoma and intraocular pressure distribution in a defined population: the Egna-Neumarkt Study. Ophthalmology. 1998;105(2):209–15.

5. Momont AC, Mills RP. Glaucoma screening: current perspectives and future directions. Semin Ophthalmol. 2013;28(3):185–90.

6. Bock R, Meier J, Nyiil LG, Hornegger J, Michelson G. Glaucoma risk index: automated glaucoma detection from color fundus images. Med Image Anal. 2010;14(3):471–81.

7. Patton N, Aslam TM, MacGillivray T, Deary IJ, Dhillon B, Eikelboom RH, et al. Retinal image analysis: concepts, applications and potential. Prog Retin Eye Res. 2006;25(1):99–127.

8. Budai A, Odstrčilik J. High resolution fundus image database. 2013. Available from: http://www5.cs.fau.de/research/data/fundus-images.

9. Nayak J, Acharya UR, Bhat PS, Shetty N, Lim TC. Automated diagnosis of glaucoma using digital fundus images. J Med Syst. 2008;33(5):337–46.

10. Kruse F, Burk R, Völcker H, Zinser G, Harbarth U. Reproducibility of topographic measurements of the optic nerve head with laser tomographic scanning. Ophthalmology. 1989;96(9):1320–4.

11. Swindale NV, Stjepanovic G, Chin A, Mikelberg FS. Automated analysis of normal and glaucomatous optic nerve head topography images. Invest Ophthalmol Vis Sci. 2000;41(7):1730–42.

12. Huang D, Swanson EA, Lin CP, Schuman JS, Stinson WG, Chang W, et al. Optical coherence tomography. Science. 1991;254(5035):1178–81.

13. Huang ML, Chen HY. Development and comparison of automated classifiers for glaucoma diagnosis using Stratus optical coherence tomography. Invest Ophthalmol Vis Sci. 2005;46(11):4121–9.

14. Burgansky-Eliash Z, Wollstein G, Chu T, Ramsey JD, Glymour C, Noecker RJ, et al. Optical coherence tomography machine learning classifiers for glaucoma detection: a preliminary study. Invest Ophthalmol Vis Sci. 2005;46(11):4147–52.

15. Bishop CM. Pattern recognition and machine learning (information science and statistics). Secaucus: Springer-Verlag New York, Inc.; 2006.

16. Niemeijer M, Abràmoff MD, Van Ginneken B. Image structure clustering for image quality verification of color retina images in diabetic retinopathy screening. Med Image Anal. 2006;10(6):888–98.

17. Köhler T, Budai A, Kraus MF, Odstrcilik J, Michelson G, Hornegger J. Automatic no-reference quality assessment for retinal fundus images using vessel segmentation. In: IEEE 26th international symposium on Computer-Based Medical Systems (CBMS). Porto; 2013. p. 95–100.

18. Paulus J, Meier J, Bock R, Hornegger J, Michelson G. Automated quality assessment of retinal fundus photos. Int J Comput Assist Radiol Surg. 2010;5(6):557–64.

19. Abràmoff MD, Garvin MK, Sonka M. Retinal imaging and image analysis. IEEE Reviews in Biomedical Engineering. 2010;3:169–208.

20. Kubecka L, Jan J, Kolar R. Retrospective illumination correction of retinal images. Int J Biomed Imaging. 2010;2010:1–10.

21. Köhler T, Hornegger J, Mayer M, Michelson G. Quality-guided denoising for low-cost fundus imaging. In: Bildverarbeitung für die Medizin 2012. Berlin-Heidelberg: Springer; 2012. p. 292–7.

22. Meier J, Bock R, Michelson G, Nyl LG, Hornegger J. Effects of preprocessing eye fundus images on appearance based glaucoma classification. In: 12th international conference on Computer Analysis of Images and Patterns, CAIP. Lecture Notes in Computer Science (LNCS) 4673, vol. 4673/2007. Vienna; 2007. p. 165–73.

23. Joshi GD, Sivaswamy J, Krishnadas S. Optic disk and cup segmentation from monocular color retinal images for glaucoma assessment. IEEE Trans Med Imaging. 2011;30(6):1192–205.

24. Yin F, Liu J, Wong DWK, Tan NM, Cheung C, Baskaran M, et al. Automated segmentation of optic disc and optic cup in fundus images for glaucoma diagnosis. In: 2012 25th IEEE international symposium on Computer-Based Medical Systems (CBMS). IEEE Rome; 2012. p. 1–6.

25. Cheng J, Liu J, Xu Y, Yin F, Wong DWK, Tan NM, et al. Superpixel classification based optic disc and optic cup segmentation for glaucoma screening. IEEE Trans Med Imaging. 2013;32(6):1019–32.

26. Michelson G, Wärntges S, Hornegger J, Lausen B. The papilla as screening parameter for early diagnosis of glaucoma. Dtsch Arztebl Int. 2008;105(34–35):583–9.

27. Sharma P, Sample PA, Zangwill LM, Schuman JS. Diagnostic tools for glaucoma detection and management. Surv Ophthalmol. 2008;53 Suppl 1:S17–32.

28. Horn FK, Mardin CY, Laemmer R, Baleanu D, Juenemann AM, Kruse FE, et al. Correlation between local glaucomatous visual field defects and loss of nerve fiber layer thickness measured with polarimetry and spectral domain OCT. Invest Ophthalmol Vis Sci. 2009;50(5):1971–7.

29. Muramatsu C, Nakagawa T, Sawada A, Hatanaka Y, Yamamoto T, Fujita H. Automated determination of cup-to-disc ratio for classification of glaucomatous and normal eyes on stereo retinal fundus images. J Biomed Opt. 2011;16(9):096009.

30. Hancox ODMD. Optic disc size, an important consideration in the glaucoma evaluation. Clin Eye Vision Care. 1999;11(2):59–62.

31. Fayers T, Strouthidis NG, Garway-Heath DF. Monitoring glaucomatous progression using a novel Heidelberg Retina Tomograph event analysis. Ophthalmology. 2007;114(11):1973–80.

32. Twa MD, Parthasarathy S, Johnson CA, Bullimore MA. Morphometric analysis and classification of glaucomatous optic neuropathy using radial polynomials. J Glaucoma. 2012;21(5):302–12.

33. Mayer M, Borsdorf A, Wagner M, Hornegger J, Mardin CY, Tornow RP. Wavelet denoising of multiframe optical coherence tomography data. Biomed Optics Expr. 2012;3(3):572–89.

34. Salinas HM, Fernandez DC. Comparison of PDE-based nonlinear diffusion approaches for image enhancement and denoising in optical coherence tomography. IEEE Trans Med Imaging. 2007; 26(6):761–71.

35. Ozcan A, Bilenca A, Desjardins AE, Bouma BE, Tearney GJ. Speckle reduction in optical coherence tomography images using digital filtering. J Opt Soc Am A Opt Image Sci Vis. 2007;24(7):1901–10.

36. Kraus M, Potsaid B, Mayer M, Bock R, Baumann B, Liu JJ, et al. Motion correction in optical coherence tomography volumes on a per A-scan basis using orthogonal scan patterns. Biomed Optics Expr. 2012;3(6):1182–99.

37. Pachiyappan A, Das UN, Murthy TV, Tatavarti R. Automated diagnosis of diabetic retinopathy and glaucoma using fundus and OCT images. Lipids Health Dis. 2012;11:73.

38. Bizios D, Heijl A, Hougaard JL, Bengtsson B. Machine learning classifiers for glaucoma diagnosis based on classification of retinal nerve fibre layer thickness parameters measured by Stratus OCT. Acta Ophthalmol. 2010;88(1):44–52.

39. Mayer MA, Hornegger J, Mardin CY, Kruse FE, P TR. Automated glaucoma classification using nerve fiber layer segmentations on circular spectral domain OCT b-scans. The Association for Research in Vision and Ophthalmology, Inc. (ARVO) (Annual Meeting), E-Abstract. 2009.

40. Mayer MA, Hornegger J, Mardin CY, Tornow RP. Retinal nerve fiber layer segmentation on FD-OCT scans of normal subjects and glaucoma patients. Biomed Optics Expr. 2010;1(5):1358.

41. Acharya UR, Dua S, Du X, Sree SV, Chua CK. Automated diagnosis of glaucoma using texture and higher order spectra features. IEEE Trans Inf Technol Biomed. 2011;15(3):449–55.

42. Dua S, Acharya UR, Chowriappa P, Sree SV. Wavelet-based energy features for glaucomatous image classi-fication. IEEE Trans Inf Technol Biomed. 2012;16(1):80–7.

43. Turk M, Pentland A. Eigenfaces for recognition. J Cogn Neurosci. 1991;3(1):71–86.

44. Fink F, Worle K, Gruber P, Tome A, Gorriz-Saez J, Puntonet C, et al. ICA analysis of retina images for glaucoma classification. In: Engineering in Medicine and Biology Society, 2008. EMBS 2008. 30th annual international conference of the IEEE. IEEE Vancouver; 2008. p. 4664–7.

45. Hyvärinen A, Oja E. Independent component analysis: algorithms and applications. Neural Netw. 2000;13(4):411–30.

10

Yuliya Naumchuk, Vinay A. Shah, and Simon Kaja

Contents

Y. Naumchuk, BS
Department of Ophthalmology, Vision Research
Center, University of Missouri-Kansas City School
of Medicine, 2411 Holmes St., Kansas City,
MO 64108, USA

V.A. Shah, MD
Department of Ophthalmology, Dean McGee Eye
Institute, University of Oklahoma,
608 Stanton L. Young Blvd., Oklahoma City,
OK 73104, USA

S. Kaja, PhD (✉)
Department of Ophthalmology, Vision Research
Center, University of Missouri-Kansas City School
of Medicine, 2411 Holmes St., Kansas City,
MO 64108, USA

K&P Scientific LLC, Corporate Office,
8570 N Hickory St.
Ste. 412, Kansas City, MO 64155, USA
e-mail: kajas@umkc.edu, kaja@kpsci.com

10.1   Mobile Technology in Tele-education

10.1.1 Definition and Terms

Tele-medicine is defined as "the use of medical information exchanged from one site to another via electronic communications to improve, maintain, or assist patients' health status" [1]. As such, tele-medicine includes electronic health, telehealth, telematics, and also tele-education [2]. Over the past decades, tele-medicine and tele-education, in particular, have seen a dramatic change as physicians and educators have embraced novel technology. Long gone are the days of distributing DVRs: educational programs are now available online, either as scheduled live web conferencing (webinars) or on-demand. The main advantages of tele-education are increased flexibility, increased capacity for educational institutions compared with traditional learning, and uniform distribution of educational material outside academic centers [2].

Tremendous advances in the field of mobile communication over the past decade have contributed significantly to both the availability and

G. Michelson (ed.), *Teleophthalmology in Preventive Medicine*,
DOI 10.1007/978-3-662-44975-2_10, © Springer-Verlag Berlin Heidelberg 2015

popularity of tele-education, largely as a direct result of the advent of the smartphone allowing content to be downloaded through the network carrier data service while on the go. The Oxford English Dictionary defines a smartphone as "a cellular phone that is able to perform many of the functions of a computer, typically having a relatively large screen and an operating system capable of running general-purpose applications" [3].

10.1.2 History

The first smartphone was first introduced by IBM in 1993, even although at that time the term smartphone had not yet been coined. IBM's "Simon" was the most advanced and high-tech cell phone of its time, featuring emailing capabilities, a calendar, world clock, fax function, a calculator, and games, all controlled through a touch screen interface. Some of the early smartphones included Nokia's 9000, launched in 1996, and Ericsson's R380, which was released in the year 2000. It was in fact the concept version for the R380, named "GS 88 Penelope," which was called a "Smart Phone." Research in Motion Inc. released their 6000 series Blackberry in 2003, which dominated the global smartphone market for the following 5 years. Earlier Java-based Blackberry models had cell phone capabilities but required a headphone for cellular communication. Rapidly, future models evolved to include color screens, Bluetooth™ capability, integrated speakerphones, global positioning system (GPS), a camera, trackball interface support, internal memory cards, and additional software, marking the start of a transition from devices primarily targeted at businesses to consumer models. The major event in the history of smartphones was the launch of Apple's iPhone in January 2007, which started a transformation of the perception of cellular and mobile communication, which is perhaps best summarized by a quote attributed to Steve Jobs, CEO of Apple Inc., that "the phone was not just a communication tool but a way of life." With the ability to run third-party software applications, so-called apps, available through Apple's iTunes Store, the iPhone truly deserved

the name "smart phone" and revolutionized the cellular communications market (see Fig. 10.1). The first Android operating system phone, the HTC Dream, was then released on the US market in 2008, 2 years prior to the first Google phone. A comprehensive up-to-date history and perspective on smartphones is given in [4]. Today, it is estimated that approximately 50 % of the general population in the USA and more than 95 % of US physicians own a smartphone, and smartphones have become an integral part of our daily lives for work, study, and play.

10.1.3 Today

Today's smartphone market is dominated by two players, Apple Inc. and Google Inc., who combine 92.3 % of all smartphone operating system shipments in the first quarter of 2013 [5]. While Android had a 75 % market share, iOS contributed 17.3 % to the total operating system shipments, with Windows Phone and Blackberry OS making up 3.2 and 2.9 %, respectively, according to the same study. However, despite the dominance by Android overall, the healthcare sector remains strongly dominated by Apple. While it is notoriously difficult to accurately determine mobile communication hardware preferences, estimates suggest that almost 90 % of physicians use and prefer Apple mobile devices over Android or any of the other competitors. Why? Several reasons are likely the cause for this very uneven distribution compared with the general public:

1. Apps. There is a much larger number of high-quality medical applications for the Apple platform compared with Android (cf. 6).
2. Integration. Apple has maintained a strong position by integrating several devices, and many apps work on both the iPhone and Apple's iPad or have even been converted to dedicated tablet versions.
3. Compatibility. Apple provides iOS updates for most supported devices ensuring that apps continue to work. In contrast, there are multiple versions of the Android OS on the market and not all apps work seamlessly with all the versions.

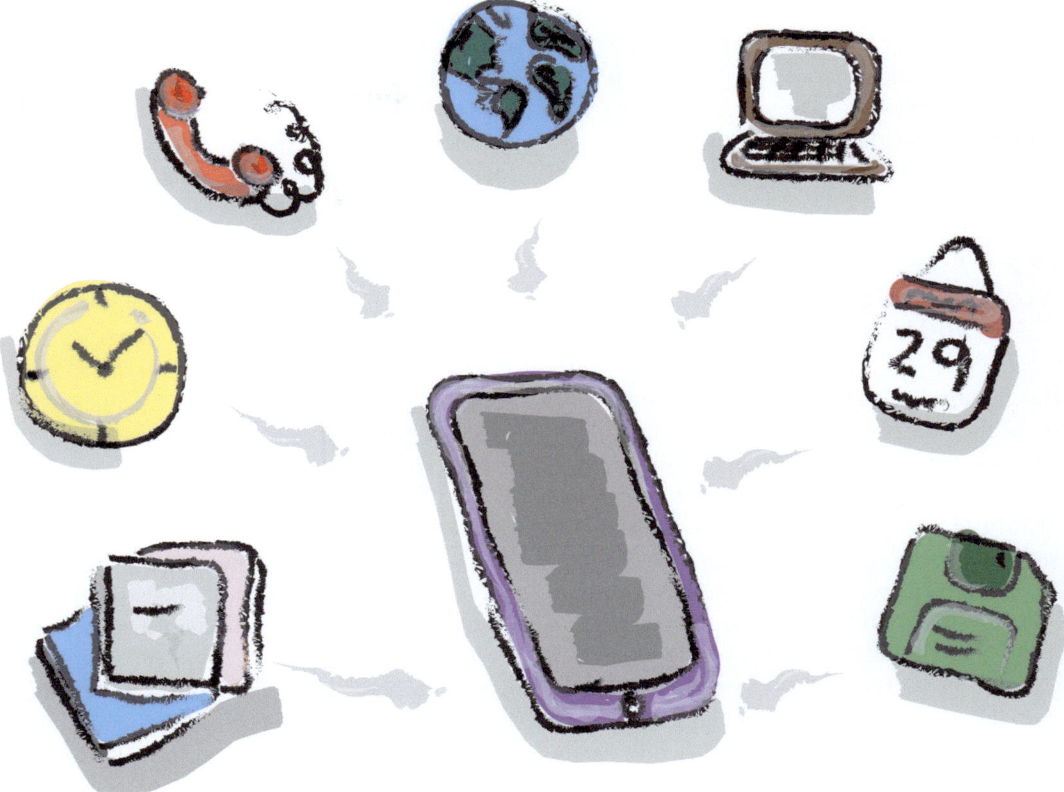

Fig. 10.1 The smartphone has changed our lives and also the healthcare profession. Office-based tasks can now be completed "on the go," and the smartphone has taken the place of reference books, the desk phone, stationary Internet computers, and handheld assistants (Illustration: Joe Moran, UMKC School of Medicine)

4. Implementation. Many academic institutions have implemented Apple hardware, notably iPads, into their education curricula as well as patient care. Apple's strength in integration clearly has swayed the decision making of healthcare professionals and educators toward choosing an iPhone over an Android-based smartphone.

What does the future hold? In the short history of mobile phones and smartphones, no single player has dominated the market both in terms of technological innovation and market share for more than 5–6 years. Research in Motion has begun a major restructuring of the company and recently released 4G LTE-compatible devices, the BlackBerry Q10 and Z10 smartphones, as well as their BlackBerry PlayBook tablet. It remains to be seen whether the BlackBerry™ will have its comeback. Nonetheless, industry-leading security standards and exceptional email integration remain the most important purchase decision factors for a BlackBerry device. Furthermore, BlackBerry sales may benefit from new regulations and privacy concerns regarding the security of medical records.

Software applications, *apps*, are available through application distribution platforms based on the mobile operating system. For iPhones and iPad, apps are available through the Apple App Store, while Android apps are distributed via the Google Play. Microsoft and Research in Motion operate the Windows Phone Store and BlackBerry App World, respectively. Many apps, including specialized medical apps, are free, while others are offered for purchase (in the medical field often the case for reference works and textbooks) or on a subscription model. In the following, we will describe some of the various types of apps available for ophthalmologists.

10.2 Apps and Tools for the Ophthalmologist and Vision Researcher

The number of apps specifically designed for the healthcare provider is rapidly growing, and there are countless apps with an ophthalmological focus [6, 7]. Recent studies have shown that up to a third of physicians make prescription decisions based on data from smartphone apps [8]. However, with patient safety in mind, assessing the quality, accuracy, and currentness of the content makes choosing an app far from a simple task. The larger the number of apps used for medical decision making, the greater the time and effort required to update the apps, organize the device, and remember "which is which." This also means that an app that incorporates as many features into one application as possible and at the same time maintains a user-friendly and logical interface will provide the greatest gain in productivity.

The one single most comprehensive app on the market, available for both iPhone and Android, is the *Eye Handbook*. *Eye Handbook* was originally launched for iPhone in 2009 and has since had more than 750,000 downloads and updates, making it the most popular ophthalmological smartphone app.

10.2.1 The Eye Handbook

The *Eye Handbook* (Cloud 9 Development, LLC) was developed by ophthalmologists for ophthalmologists and features the most comprehensive collection of tools for ophthalmological testing as well as patient and physician education.

The *Eye Handbook* is a free application that is currently available in the iTunes and Google Play Stores.

The included testing tools such as near vision cards, color vision plates (see Fig. 10.2), animated pediatric fixation targets, Amsler grids, etc. (for complete listing, see Table 10.1), will of course not replace office-based testing under ideal conditions; however, these tools can be particularly useful in the clinical setting when performing inpatient consults and emergency room visits. An additional advantage is their use in rural areas and in assisted living facilities, where office visits often pose a significant strain and burden on patients.

One important aspect in the daily clinical practice is patient education. Providing verbal, visual, or written material to improve patient understanding of ophthalmic diseases and disease processes is a critical factor for successful treatment approaches as well as compliance. *Eye Handbook* provides a plethora of patient resources, which include a 3D rendering of a rotating eyeball allowing the physician to delineate specific anatomical considerations in medical or surgical disease management. Also included is a list of the most common disease processes encountered in the day-to-day ophthalmology practice. Short, succinct narratives provide relevant and credible patient education, including links to several third-party website with informative content. A section for coding provides ICD-9, CPT codes, and a special section for commonly used modifiers in ophthalmology. This provides an easy-to-use always-available coding resource for the practicing physician. The newly launched Media Center and Forums sections provide various educational tools (flash cards, surgical videos, and lectures) and the opportunity to share and discuss complicated cases with colleagues. Various medical and ophthalmological calculators are also included (see Fig. 10.2).

At this time, the Eye Handbook is the most comprehensive and up-to-date ophthalmology app available for iPhone and Android [6, 7]. The

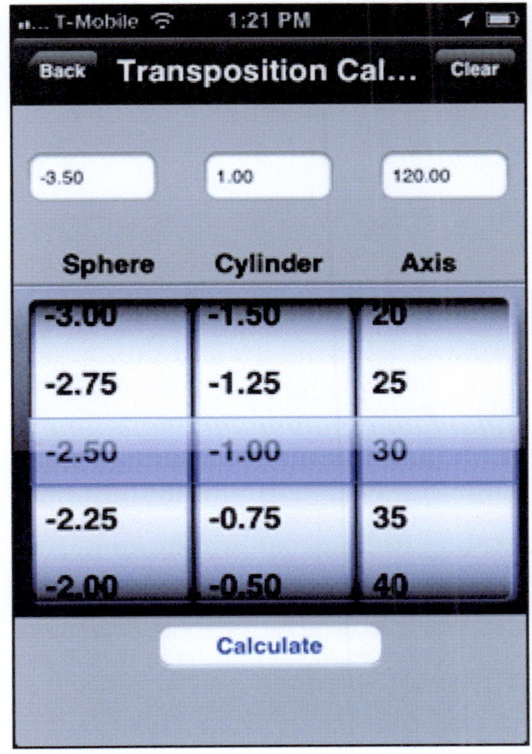

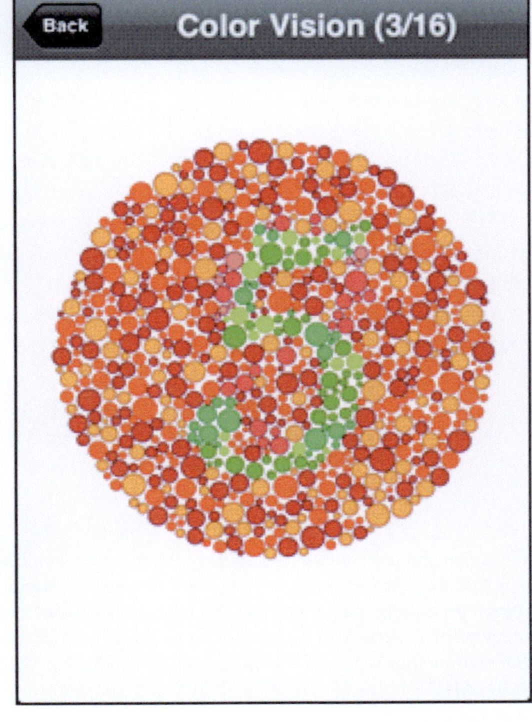

Fig. 10.2 Screenshots from the Eye Handbook app. *Left*: The transposition calculator is one many calculator tools available in the application. *Right*: Color vision slide to diagnose colorblindness (Reproduction of screenshots with permission by Cloud Nine Development, LLC)

Eye Handbook is offered as a free app through the Apple iTunes Store for iOS and the Google Play Store for Android OS.

10.2.2 Atlas of Ophthalmology

The Atlas of Ophthalmology app is the iPhone version of the online-based Atlas of Ophthalmology. A pictorial documentation of eye disease, the emphasis of the Atlas is placed on highlighting the clinical manifestations and various stages through around 2,500 photographs and ancillary tests, rather than by providing a detailed overview of disease pathophysiology, diagnosis, and treatment. The Atlas is offered free of charge as long as it is used for educational purposes.

10.2.3 Epocrates Rx

Besides specialized ophthalmological apps, there are a number of general medical apps, which also can prove useful to the ophthalmologist. Epocrates Rx is a free drug reference app that provides up-to-date information on drugs and drug interactions. The information on drugs includes search functionalities for generic and trade names and information on adult and pediatric dosing. Each entry also provides details on adverse effects, drug interactions, and black box warnings as well as the pharmacological profile of the drug. The app also provides estimated retail drug pricing for patients and information regarding the coverage/reimbursement by a large number of US insurance plans.

Table 10.1 Features available in the *Eye Handbook* app

Calculators	Testing	Other features
Age to bifocal add	Accommodation test	Coding
Amplitude of accommodation	Amsler grids	Equipment
Diopter to radius conversion	Color vision	Eye atlas
Glaucoma risk calculator	Contrast sensitivity test	EHB manual
IOL calculators	Duochrome test	Meds
IOP–CCT calculator	Fluorescein light	References
SIAC	Near vision cards	RSS feeds
Toric calculators	Near vision cards (inverted)	Treatment
Transposition calculator	OKN drum	*Patient tools*
Vertex conversion	Peds fixation targets	Eye diagrams
Visual acuity calculator	Peds optotypes	Media consent form
	Penlight	Patient education
	Pupil gauge	Vision symptoms
	Red screen bilateral	
	Red screen unilateral	
	Ruler	
	Worth 4 dot	

Physician and patient tools available in the *Eye Handbook* app. The app offers a large number of calculators and tools that can facilitate eye exams in the non-office setting. The Media Consent form allows the patient to sign a release right on the screen permitting the publication and educational use of audio, video, and photography, as well as sharing the media with other medical personnel for consultation. The consent form can be emailed directly and can be stored on the device
IOL intraocular lens, *CCT* central corneal thickness, *SIAC* Surgically Induced Astigmatism Calculator, *OKN* optokinetic, *EHB* Eye Handbook, *RSS* Rich Site Summary

Epocrates Rx also contains a number of useful reference features. Pill ID not only provides an image of a given drug and a detailed description of the pill characteristics, it also allows identifying a pill based on its physical characteristics (such as color or shape) and/or the imprint code. Helping patients identify the correct pills or ensuring that medications are sufficiently different for patients to easily distinguish can help prevent medication errors, which are frequently associated with serious consequences.

10.2.4 Clinical Trial Information

Clinical trial information is also available at the fingertip, and a growing number of apps feature access to clinical trial databases. The app *Clinical Trials* (StopWatch Media Inc., Philadelphia, PA, USA) mines databases by the National Library of Medicine and National Institutes of Health to list over 86,000 clinical trials registered with the US government. Access to the information is provided by means of an intuitive search interface with search options and limiters similar to the regular web interface. Advanced search options in the *Clinical Trials* app include searching for type trial (observational, interventional, or expanded access), location, clinical trial phase, and enrolment status. Various email features within the app are designed for emailing both individual trial information and an entire list of relevant trials using the iPhone's email interface, allowing easy sharing of the information with patients and colleagues. Furthermore, the app has customizable email templates for contacting the study coordinator and principal investigators with questions regarding the trial.

10.2.5 Wills Eye Manual and Other Reference Resources

Various time-tested references are now available in the mobile format and e-books. *Wills Eye Manual* is available on a yearly subscription basis. Various other ophthalmology textbooks are also now available on a number of different purchase or subscription models. Similarly, most peer-reviewed ophthalmology journals can be accessed through their respective apps or a smartphone-friendly website interface.

10.2.6 Tools for Vision Research

Over the past years, the presence of smartphones in the basic science laboratory has significantly increased. Especially popular among younger students and research staff, the smartphone has replaced timers, calculators, and other small digital aids. Moreover, the number of specialized basic science applications has steadily increased over recent years. Again, estimating the number of scientific apps is difficult to estimate, mostly as many apps currently available may be categorized as reference, medical, productivity, or utility app.

More recently, many manufacturers now also provide iPhone or Android apps as product support. While some of these are mere smartphone versions of websites or online catalogs, others include technical references and animated tutorials for a variety of equipment and consumables used in a modern vision research laboratory.

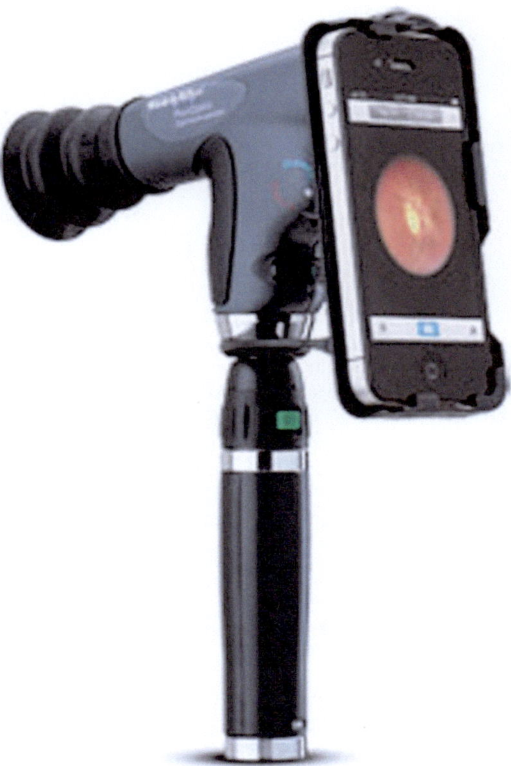

Fig. 10.3 The Welch Allyn iExaminer turns the iPhone into a high-resolution imaging device for fundus and retinal nerve (Photo with permission from Welch Allyn Inc.)

10.3 The Smartphone as a Device for Research and Diagnostics

Technological advances have turned the smartphone in a powerful computer that can compete with laptops and stationary computers, and computing capabilities have surpassed the microchips in small handheld research and diagnostic devices. Most recently, a number of devices have appeared on the market that utilize the smartphone, in most cases the iPhone, as the portable hardware, computing, or image acquisition backbone.

10.3.1 iExaminer

Welch Allyn Inc. (Skaneateles Falls, NY) recently launched the iExaminer add-on, which turns their market-leading PanOptic Ophthalmoscope into a smartphone-powered digital imaging device (see Fig. 10.3). Using an adaptor that aligns the optical access of the PanOptic Ophthalmoscope to the visual axis of the iPhone camera allows the capture of high-resolution pictures of the fundus and retinal nerve. Images are acquired and saved using the iExaminer app. Featuring the unique field of view of the PanOptic Ophthalmoscope, which provides a five times larger fundus view than a typical ophthalmoscope and a 25° field of view without the need for dilating the pupil, the iExaminer allows fundus imaging in the non-office setting. Of particular note, the iExaminer has received 501(K) FDA clearance. It is anticipated that such an inexpensive solution will enable screening for ocular disorders in the primary care or non-office setting, especially for the prevention or early diagnosis of diabetic retinopathy.

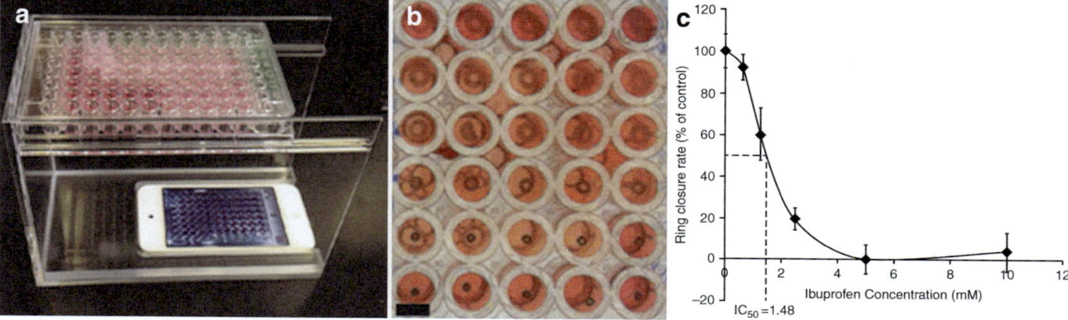

Fig. 10.4 (**a**) The mobile device-based imaging setup of the BiO-ring closure assay. The 96-well plate is placed on the top of the setup. The smartphone device is located at the bottom of the setup, with the camera facing upward to image the whole plate. (**b**) A sample image taken with the mobile device of 30 rings of HEK293s and ibuprofen. Note the dark color and the resolution of the rings within the media. Scale bar: 5 mm. (**c**) Dose–response curve of ibuprofen and HEK293s resulting from the analysis of changes in ring diameter measured from images shown in (b) as a function of time. The rate of ring closure was found by fitting diameter–time curves using linear least-squares fits and then normalizing the rates to control. The IC_{50} was found to be 1.48 mM. Error bars represent standard deviation (figure with permission from n3D Biosciences Inc., Houston, TX)

10.3.2 The BiO-Ring Closure Assay

The BiO-ring closure assay (n3D Biosciences Inc., Houston, TX) uses an iPhone/iPod in combination with their proprietary 3D cell culturing technology using the magnetic levitation method. In this configuration, the mobile device is used for image capture (see Fig. 10.4a) of cells migrating in a 3D cell culturing environment. In this assay, the rate of migration can be used to generate dose–dependence curves for measuring drug toxicity or efficacy, as shown in the case for ibuprofen, a known nephrotoxic drug, and exposure on human embryonic kidney (HEK-293) cells (see Fig. 10.4b, c). The use of the smartphone device allows for compact and environmental experiments to be performed with standard cell culturing incubators while forgoing the need for large and expensive imaging equipment such as microscopes. The dark brown color of the nanoparticles and the density of the 3D culture in this system allow distinguishing the 3D culture and provide contrast against the surrounding media. Commonly available mobile devices have cameras with sufficient resolution to capture whole plates rather than individual wells, and these mobile devices can be programmed to take images at specific time points. This method eliminates the need to image cultures under a microscope at multiple time points, which reduces the risk of contamination from moving plates in and out of sterile environments.

10.3.3 Other Devices

Over the past year, a growing number of iPhone-powered medical and diagnostic devices have been launched. These include adapters for slit lamps (Slit Lamp iPhone Adapter by Optivision2020, Inc.), probe adapters for measuring blood glucose levels (iBGStar by Sanofi-Aventis LLC), and even connections for mobile ultrasound diagnostics (MobiUS™SP1 by MobiSante Inc.). The number of such devices is likely to grow exponentially over the coming years, especially given the endorsement and approval by the FDA for mobile solutions that can assist prophylaxis and early diagnosis of a number of devastating disorders of societal importance.

Conclusions

Over the past decade, we have witnessed a revolutionary change in the field of medicine: tele-education and tele-medicine have become omnipresent, as cell phones have developed into high-end portable computers. While early smartphones provided email access and limited browser capabilities, large multimedia file downloads in high-definition (HD) quality are now possible and, more importantly, extremely fast, as carrier network data speeds match or even exceed the average data transfer rate of a home DSL service. Furthermore, memory and storage have increased such that a practically unlimited number of software applications can be downloaded to the latest generation of smartphones. Most apps are offered free or for a modest fee and can be installed on multiple devices, which has led to a healthy competition between app developers and prevented market dominance previously seen with standard office software for desktop computers.

Perhaps one of the biggest questions in recent years was whether the smartphone would increase productivity or simply add distraction. Productivity apps certainly now seamlessly integrate all sources of information, and high data speeds and availability of network data services and public and corporate WiFi hotspots provide for the continuous synchronization of files between office computers, cloud servers, and the smartphone. Dictation tools and smart touch input allow "typing" at similar speeds as on a regular, full-size keyboard and make the tedious input using the number keyboard on a small cellular phone a distant memory. Professional apps, such as the *Eye Handbook* presented above, now also increase our productivity in the clinical and laboratory setting, by providing a single tool to assist with patient education, clinical testing and diagnostics, reference works, and much more. Similarly, using the smartphone as medical or diagnostic device, data is available immediately for wireless synchronization and dissemination. So overall, the smartphone certainly has the capabilities to make us more productive and efficient, when utilizing available tools to their maximum extent. However, education on efficient smartphone use is necessary to fully utilize the benefits it offers, much similar to the early computer courses in the early days of the digital age.

Otherwise, smartphones will remain an expensive gadget for recreational use.

Acknowledgments Generous support by the University of Missouri, Kansas City, Department of Ophthalmology and Vision Research Center is gratefully acknowledged. SK would like to thank the BlackBerry® Academic Program for supporting his research program on smartphone applications in ophthalmology.

Financial Disclosures

YN: none
VS: Dr. Shah is cofounder of Cloud 9 Development, LLC, and the co-developer of the Eye Handbook app.
SK: none

References

1. The American Telemedicine Association. Core standards for telemedicine operations. ATA standards & guidelines [Internet]. 2007 [cited 16 May 2013]. Available from: http://www.americantelemed.org/docs/default-source/standards/core-standards-for-telemedicine-operations.pdf..
2. Masic I, Pandza H, Kulasin I, Masic Z, Valjevac S. Tele-education as method of medical education. Med Arh. 2009;63(6):350–3.
3. Smartphone [Internet]. Oxford University Press. 2013 [cited 16 May 2013]. Available from: http://oxforddictionaries.com/us/definition/american_english/smartphone.
4. Taplin B. Smartphone history: evolution & revolution [monograph online]. 2013 [cited 16 May 2013]. Available from: Amazon Digital Services, Inc.
5. Android and iOS combine for 92.3 % of all smartphone operating system shipments in the first quarter while windows phone leapfrogs BlackBerry, According to IDC [Internet]. 2013 [cited 16 May 2013]. Available from: http://www.idc.com/getdoc.jsp?containerId=prUS24108913.
6. Chhablani J, Kaja S, Shah VA. Smartphones in ophthalmology. Indian J Ophthalmol. 2012;60(2):127–31.
7. Lord RK, Shah VA, San Filippo AN, Krishna R. Novel uses of smartphones in ophthalmology. Ophthalmology. 2010;117(6):1274–e3.
8. Alvarez A. How are physicians using smartphones for professional purposes? [Internet] 2013 [cited 16 May 2013]. Available from: http://www.kantarmedia-healthcarecom/how-are-physicians-using-smartphones-for-professional-purposes.

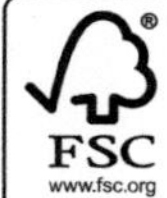